Praise for *Yoga Where You Are*

"In *Yoga Where You Are*, Dianne Bondy and Kat Heagberg offer indispensable knowledge for all yoga practitioners to personalize their practice and honor the body they're in today. This book is a much-needed resource for yoga students in bigger bodies, stiff bodies, older bodies, and disabled bodies since many teachers don't know how to work with us. Now we can take our practice back into our own hands. I can't wait to share this excellent resource in my teacher trainings and with my students."

—AMBER KARNES, founder of Body Positive Yoga

"*Yoga Where You Are* is a resource for all people to practice in a way that meets them where they are . . . and grow with them! It offers the opportunity to learn, explore, and practice with an emphasis on accessibility, creative variations, and a message deeply rooted in self-acceptance and a celebration of the worth and value of all bodies, all people. I highly recommend this as a foundational yoga book for anyone and everyone at any point on their yoga journey."

—MELANIE KLEIN, cofounder of the Yoga & Body Image Coalition, editor of *Yoga Rising: 30 Empowering Stories from Yoga Renegades for Every Body*

"In an industry where the phrase 'we're all one' is far too often used to dismiss, marginalize, and exclude those who don't fit the thin, flexible, able, white-bodied mold, this book is a revelation! Dianne and Kat speak to a shared humanity that isn't about sameness but rather about celebrating our differences so that everyone can experience the benefits that yoga can offer."

—JESAL PARIKH, co-host of the *Yoga Is Dead* podcast

"The future of yoga looks like this—people of all abilities sharing a practice that is designed to connect us to a deeper part of ourselves and to each other. Yoga has the power to transform our lives personally as well as collectively, but that can only happen when we share a practice that is designed to be welcoming for all. Dianne Bondy and Kat Heagberg have shown us how to do that in a masterful and yet simple way."

—JIVANA HEYMAN, author of *Accessible Yoga*

YOGA WHERE YOU ARE

CUSTOMIZE YOUR PRACTICE FOR YOUR BODY + YOUR LIFE

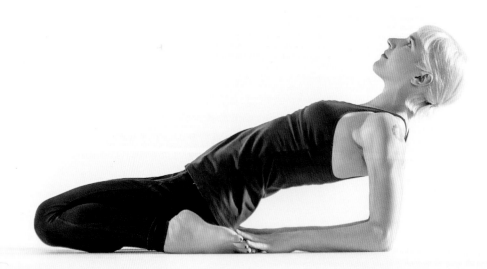

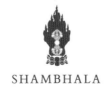

DIANNE BONDY +
KAT HEAGBERG

FOREWORD BY JES BAKER
PHOTOS BY ANDREA KILLAM

SHAMBHALA

Shambhala Publications, Inc.
4720 Walnut Street
Boulder, Colorado 80301
www.shambhala.com

© 2020 by Dianne Bondy and Kat Heagberg
All photos by Andrea Killam

Cover photos: Andrea Killam
Cover design: Alex Hennig
Interior design: Laura Shaw Design

9 8 7 6 5 4 3 2 1

First Edition
Printed in China

⊗ This edition is printed on acid-free paper that meets the American National Standards Institute
Z39.48 Standard.
♻ Shambhala Publications makes every effort to print on recycled paper.
For more information please visit www.shambhala.com.
Shambhala Publications is distributed worldwide by Penguin Random House, Inc., and its subsidiaries.

Library of Congress Cataloging-in-Publication Data

Names: Bondy, Dianne, author. | Heagberg, Kat, author.
Title: Yoga where you are: customize your practice for your body and your life / Dianne Bondy and
    Kat Heagberg.
Description: First edition. | Boulder, Colorado: Shambhala, 2020. | Includes bibliographical references
    and index.
Identifiers: LCCN 2019053634 | ISBN 9781611807868 (trade paperback)
Subjects: LCSH: Hatha yoga. | Yoga.
Classification: LCC RA781.7.B66124 2020 | DDC 613.7/046—dc23
LC record available at https://lccn.loc.gov/2019053634

Contents

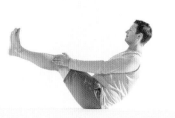

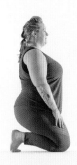

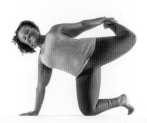

List of Poses

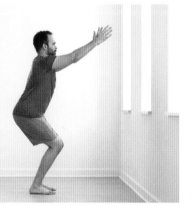
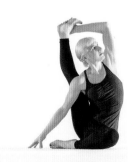
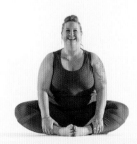

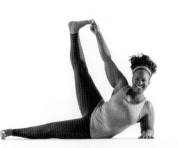

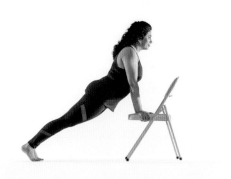

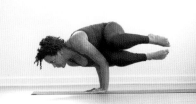

Foreword

Jes Baker

As someone who lives in a fat body and believes that every person deserves the opportunity to move in the body they have (however they like), I have seen the struggle for a lot of us to reclaim the physical part of ourselves that society is quick to "other." As a fat-positive body liberationist, it is my mission to change the current narrative of self-hate to one of self-acceptance and ultimately, inclusive freedom. In both of my books, *Things No One Will Tell Fat Girls* and *Landwhale*, I speak about all the things that fat bodies can do if desired, including finding joy in movement, exploring love, and enjoying intimate relationships. My hope is that through these conversations and through similar conversations that other incredible world changers have been having for decades, we can all learn how to become empowered by rewriting our bodily narrative and deciding what we personally need while on our healing journey.

I see and experience *some* of the struggles for people in nonconforming bodies to find joyful movement. For a long time, fitness culture, the wellness industry (which is diet culture, but y'know, just rebranded), and specifically yoga have been influenced by the socially vetted beauty standard and diet culture. But beauty standards and diet culture tell us only one story: that thin, white, able-bodied, and conventionally attractive people are the lucky few who get to dictate and participate in their own wellness and happiness. It is this same cultural idea that has made yoga about acrobatic poses, expensive athletic wear, and other elite ideals. The reality is that while no one is obligated to move their body (*ever*), moving our bodies can be a powerful tool used to reconnect our body and brain through healing our nervous system—something that every body deserves. It seems especially important to me that those who have experienced traumatic situations through cultural oppression are also afforded access to the multitude of ways we can physically reconnect through compassionate movement. Healing is a right for all.

The yoga and wellness industry has created an image that rarely celebrates the diversity of body sizes, abilities, race, or age (among other diverse aspects) that we see around us in real life. Dianne and Kat tackle these ideas head-on. This book is about representing more people on the mat, creating clarity about what yoga is, and celebrating more options for asana and different bodies. *Yoga Where You Are* celebrates the diversity of yoga through postures, breath, and philosophy. It explores yoga through our individual experiences in the collective practice while also offering recommendations for teachers on how to create safer, more inclusive practice spaces and sequences for their students. *Yoga Where You Are* will help you gain the confidence to trust your body and find your place on the mat.

Three—no, FOUR—cheers for Dianne and Kat who have used their years of experience within the yoga world to create this phenomenal guide. This exploration of yoga allows us to move deeper into our practice while also meeting us wherever we're at when it comes to healing our connection with our body! Doing this is no small feat, and we need more of this in our world.

Introduction

Why *Yoga Where You Are?*

This book is for *you*, just as you are and just where you are. It is also the yoga book that we ourselves were craving!

IT GROWS WITH YOUR PRACTICE

We hope this book meets you where you are on your yoga journey—whether you're a beginner or seasoned practitioner—and inspires your creativity and flourishing, both on the mat and in your life! As teachers, teacher trainers, and longtime students of yoga, we've both been frustrated by the lack of comprehensive, yet approachable, yoga books available. Now, don't get us wrong; there are a *lot* of yoga books out there, but we found that many of them were either too basic or too esoteric for our needs. We wished for a book that would *grow with us*, a mat-side companion that we could turn to for years to come. We didn't want a rigid manual telling us the "right" way to practice poses. We wanted something that would spark our *own* creativity and inspire our practice and teaching as our bodies and our lives evolve.

IT CELEBRATES DIVERSITY

Yoga practitioners span ages, races and ethnicities, genders, body types, and experience levels. We want to highlight more folks in our book than you usually see represented in mainstream yoga publications. In recent years, there have been more yoga books written by and for people in larger bodies, but these books are often written specifically for (or marketed specifically to) beginners. We are also happy to see more books by teachers of color. However, in general, books for teachers and more experienced practitioners have primarily featured models that fit the young, white, slim, heteronormative "yoga image" that the media often perpetuates. We recognize that millions of people live with eating disorders (over 30 million in the United States alone, according to the National Association of Anorexia Nervosa and Associated Disorders). This is something that we have both experienced ourselves, and we see the danger in yoga teachings peppered with messages about "cleansing," "detoxing," and weight loss, which we feel are inherently harmful. That's why we created the kind of resource we want to recommend to our students and teachers-in-training—a resource that celebrates all bodies and highlights the power of yoga for everyone.

IT HIGHLIGHTS ACCESSIBILITY AS STRENGTH

The practice of yoga (asana, meditation, and more) has offered deep benefit in our lives, and we want to share these practices in a way accessible to many bodies. We share pose variations not as lesser modifications, but as wonderful options that can help a wide range of students explore postures. We use language that celebrates students making wise decisions for their bodies and their lives. We hope more students and teachers will begin to use this language for themselves. Accessibility is strength.

IT OFFERS ALIGNMENT OPTIONS FOR MANY BODIES

This is book is not full of "dos and don'ts," "always and nevers," or arbitrary rules about what a pose "should" look or feel like. The truth is, yoga "alignment rules" are often based not on safety but on aesthetic preferences. Though pose alignment is often treated as universal, throughout our combined years of study, practice, and teaching, we've come to realize that this isn't true. What is or isn't "good alignment" depends on the students: their unique physical structure, their history and experiences, and their goals and intentions. Two examples from our own lives:

> **KAT:** Staff pose (see page 129) is essentially sitting upright on the floor with legs extended forward, arms alongside the body, and hands on the floor beside the hips. The purpose of staff pose is typically to help students find a long neutral spine—to sit tall without "slumping." I have a long torso and short arms, so when I plant my hands flat on the floor beside my hips in this pose, my spine rounds, defeating the purpose of the pose. To keep my spine long, I typically press my fingertips (not my palms) into the floor or place a prop (like yoga blocks) under my hands. This allows me to experience the benefits of staff pose. But throughout my yoga life, I have had many yoga instructors—and not just inexperienced teachers—"correct" my alignment in this pose, encouraging me to plant my hands flat on the floor (even though that makes my spine round) because "that's how the pose *should* be done." I've also been assured that I will be able to plant my hands flat "when I get more flexible," which I find funny, because no matter how flexible I get, my arm bones aren't going to grow any longer!

> **DIANNE:** As a woman of color in a more substantial body, I often feel very left out of a practice that primarily caters to thinner, more athletic bodies. I find

myself in classes where I am struggling with a pose, and the teacher simply doesn't have the skill to offer assistance. Most yoga teachers are unfamiliar with working with larger bodies or bodies with disabilities. Sometimes teachers are so attached to their yoga lineage or alignment principles that they miss the opportunity to engage with their students and help them in the postures. Creating variations for poses requires some ingenuity and openness to thinking outside the lineage and our traditional training to help our students. I always say there are many ways to make potatoes and there are many ways to practice asana. Let's explore how different bodies move and incorporate those movements into the bigger picture of yoga. As a larger-bodied woman, I have had to adapt yoga poses to fit my body and in doing so have been able to share my adaptations with others. It has become my mission to make yoga practice as accessible as possible.

YOGA WHERE YOU ARE

We've been frustrated (but not surprised) to have many people come to us and say, "I picked up a book about yoga and realized that it wasn't for me." We believe that yoga really is for everybody. And we'd like to see that become more than just a slogan.

Together, we have over thirty years of combined teaching experience. We've had the great privilege of working with people practicing with disabilities, people in larger bodies, older adults, and beginners. These experiences have given us the knowledge and the confidence to make yoga practice more accessible and available to a greater number of people.

Having taught around the globe, we have learned, relearned, and unlearned a lot. Most of all, we've learned to ask questions, to be curious, and to be open to new ways of approaching the practice of yoga. Our passion and determination to create a diverse and inclusive experience within the yoga culture have taught us how to create all sorts of different variations for asana, and we're excited to share many of these variations with you here—not so you can make your practice look just like ours, but so that you can make your yoga truly your own and create a practice that truly serves your unique needs and goals. And, if you're a teacher, you can better serve the needs and goals of your students.

The first part of the book shares helpful information about yoga—celebrating its diverse roots, discussing how it intersects with body image, and introducing the basics of the practice. We'd like to thank Colin Hall, professor of religious studies and kinesiology at the University of Regina in Saskatchewan, Canada, for his support with the yoga history section.

The second part of the book shares a huge array of poses and pose variations. Whether you're a seasoned practitioner or just getting started, we hope this section will support your practice and encourage you to try something new.

The third part of the book helps you design and customize your practice from sequencing to themes.

The end of the book shares some resources we've found helpful and introduces our wonderful models.

HOW TO USE THIS BOOK

Whether you're a beginner, a seasoned yogi, or a yoga teacher, we wrote this book for *you*, to serve as a resource you can turn to at any stage of your yoga journey.

If You're a Beginner

Congratulations on your newfound endeavor! If you want to learn a little more about what this yoga thing is all about, check out the essential information in part one, including the chapters titled "Yoga Then and Now" and "Yoga, Accessibility, and Body Image." Chapter 3, "Yoga Practice Basics," has our ten tips for getting started with yoga *right now* that will help you take the first steps in establishing a customized yoga practice that meets *your* needs and goals. Chapter 4, "Breath and Drishti," gives you an opportunity to get centered and feel balanced through breathing and focus. Chapter 5 on how to use props discusses what tools might be most useful and offers ideas on common household items you can use in place of specialized props.

Part two covers the different kinds of poses and their variations, from foundational poses in chapter 6 to *savasana* variations in chapter 14. Chapter 15 covers meditation. Part three focuses on how you can design your own practice and sequences (chapter 16). A series of complete sample sequences are given in chapter 17. (We suggest starting with the "The Basics" or the "Complete Chair Practice" sequences.) You can find all of the poses described in detail—along with plenty of variations, tips, and tricks for making them your own—in the poses section.

Finally, check out "Recommended Resources" at the back of the book for our suggestions for video classes that you can take online (including classes taught by both of us!).

If You're an Experienced Practitioner

If you're looking for ways to make challenging poses work for you, or for some fun new variations, you can skip to part two. The chapters are divided by category (standing poses, arm balances, inversions, and so on) so you can easily find what you're looking for.

Or, if you want some inspiration or sequences for your home practice, you can check out the sample sequences in chapter 17 or the more customizable, outside-of-the-box ideas in the "Creative Sequencing and Customizable Vinyasa" section in chapter 16.

If You're a Teacher

We hope this book serves as a useful resource for class planning and most of all for helping your students to find fun, empowering, and accessible pose variations that work for *them*. Check out the poses section beginning with chapter 6 in part two for tons of customizable options.

We've also got your back when it comes to class planning—from sharing inspiration to getting out of a sequencing rut and trying something new. In part three, "Designing Your Practice," we've included lots of helpful resources—everything from a fill-in-the blanks sequence template to inspiring tips for designing your classes and ways to shake things up with some creative sequencing. You can also glean inspiration from our sample sequences in chapter 16.

And perhaps most important, also in chapter 16, we recommend you read "Ten Strategies for Creating a Safe Place for All." More than just about anything else, fellow teachers ask us how they can make their classes more welcoming and inclusive for all types of bodies and all levels of abilities. We answer that question and provide actionable tips that will improve your teaching and help your students feel more confident and empowered by their yoga practice.

If You're a Teacher Trainer

We know it's not easy leading teacher trainings and continuing education workshops! We've both done it. And we've often felt frustrated—trying to manage homework assignments, answering questions about the "right" way to do or teach a pose, and really working to equip our students with the tools *to teach*—to ask questions, to innovate, to improvise and not just memorize pose cues or teach from a script. That's a big reason why we created this book: to provide you with a truly useful teaching resource you can share with your teacher trainees.

Your trainees can work through all the options in the poses chapters to get the lowdown on alignment basics (including when, why, and how to break the "rules") and to get ideas and information about how to change up the "typical" form of a pose in order to better serve their students. Our hope is that they don't just explore the variations we've provided here but feel equipped to create variations of their own when the need arises.

Teacher trainees also often have tons of questions about class sequencing (and for good reason). That's why we've included practical tools that you can use to guide them in creating safe, fun, and effective class plans. These include tips for sequencing and designing a themed class, sample sequences, and more, and they can all be found in chapters 16 and 17. Chapter 16 also includes a sequence template that aspiring teachers can fill in as they begin to create their own classes.

We wish you the best on your yoga journey—wherever you are right now—and hope this book serves as a resource today and in the years become. *You've got this.*

—DIANNE AND KAT

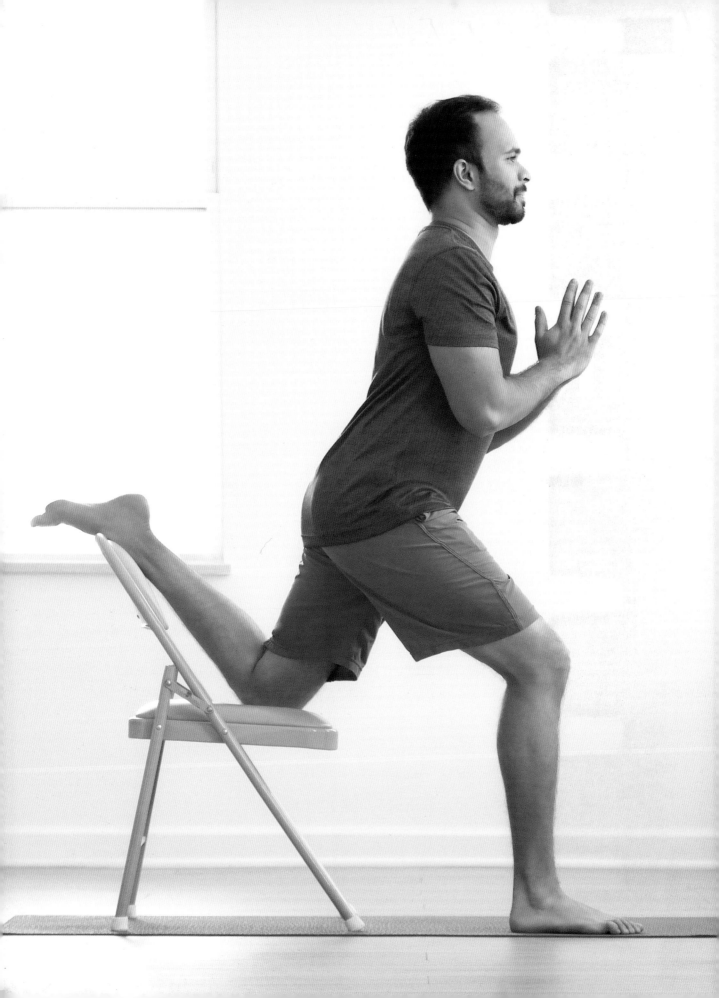

Part One **ESSENTIAL INFORMATION**

1

Yoga Then and Now

In many parts of the world, yoga has become a commodity. It is a multibillion dollar part of the fitness, wellness, and self-help industry. It has been marketed as a way to find personal transformation through ongoing, never-ending self-improvement—a scenario that, oddly enough, often promotes consumerism and a certain amount of anxiety.

We recognize the complexity of this issue as we, too, make our living in the yoga industry. According to a recent Yoga Alliance study, there are an estimated 37 million people doing yoga in the United States, yet there are likely millions more contemplating giving it a try but not feeling welcome. In order to know where we are, how we got here, and where we're going, we have to start by taking a step back. We need to understand and appreciate yoga's roots, as well as *how* yoga came to the West and how it has become a tangible commodity. By understanding this history, we can more fully embrace yoga's potential for deep change—both personally and socially.

The word *yoga* means "union" or "to yoke," to bring together. Once we realize we are all in this together, we can begin to make room for change. Yoga can be the catalyst for great change in our personal lives and in the world.

Yoga originated thousands of years ago as a vehicle for spiritual liberation, self-fulfillment, and soul evolution. Yet today it is often appropriated as a tool for beauty, fitness, or business. We want to share a history of yoga from a new perspective—one that honors its diverse roots and highlights how those of us on the margins fit in. The history of yoga is much deeper than we can share in this short chapter, but we would like to give you a taste. We hope that by honoring the roots of yoga and by emphasizing yoga's meaning of *unity* you'll be able to find new points of connection to the practice, wherever you are in your life. Yoga is evolving and will continue to evolve as humans do. Yoga has made way for many mindful movement practices that have roots and connections to this ancient practice.

YOGA AND MINDFUL MOVEMENT PRACTICES— ORIGINS AND EVOLUTION

Yoga researchers have found evidence to suggest that yoga not only originated in India but also has roots in parts of Africa, particularly Egypt. The practice of yoga was created by brown and black people as a tool for spiritual growth, as a way to integrate the spiritual element with physical experience. Over time the practice has evolved into many different forms—some more accessible than others. Today, many people have a distinct expectation of what yoga should "look like"—an expectation that often has little to no connection to yoga's roots. If we choose to look at modern yoga as a collection of mindful movements, we can see that other cultures have had an influence on yoga's history and evolution. We can, for example, see the Western influence through many accessible yoga modalities as well as the development of fitness-centered yoga.

Many different cultures created spiritual practices that connected movement and breath, whether in the form of dance, asana (postures), or exercise. One such example is Kemetic yoga.

KEMETIC YOGA

Kemetic yoga, which originated in Egypt, focuses on the movement of energy through the body in order to connect with one's higher intelligence and the divine. One practices Kemetic yoga at a much slower pace than in a standard asana class, and there is more of a focus on meditation and the chakras (energy centers). The physical poses of Kemetic yoga are taken from ancient illustrations of Egyptian gods and goddesses. It is a practice with African roots that has been largely ignored by mainstream yoga culture. This is not surprising given the history of oppression against people of African descent in North America. The contributions of people of color to modern society rarely make it into history books even though they played a huge part in the development of modern world culture.

Several preeminent researchers of Kemetic culture—particularly Sehu Khepera Ankh, St. Clair Drake, and Yirser Ra Hotep—aim to make the practice of Kemetic yoga more widely known, especially the African influence on contemporary spiritual practices. Reading about the connections between Africa and yoga has reaffirmed for Dianne that the practice was in her blood, that she fits into this culture.

Kemet, or KMT, was an ancient name for Egypt during the era of the pharaohs. Research suggests that the first Egyptians were black-skinned and came from the Sudan, Ethiopia, and southern Arabia, as well as Babylon.[1] The Kemetic people designed and built pyramids and made important contributions in many fields, including mathematics, architecture, chemistry, medicine, and more. They expressed their ideas in sacred symbols, such as those found in the pyramids and in tombs like that belonging to Tutankhamen.

Yirser Ra Hotep (also known as Elvrid Lawrence) is the most senior instructor of Kemetic yoga in the United States, with over thirty years of experience in practicing and teaching. He has written extensively on Kemetic symbols and their connections to yoga. He writes, "Through modern eyes, what these ancient people meant by their symbolic drawings and carvings appear obscure and mysterious. Through the eyes of one enlightened to their world view—their obvious and magnificent messages are easily understood."[2]

One of the examples Yirser Ra Hotep discusses involves a carving on the back of a chair found in King Tut's tomb. The carving illustrates a man called Shu. Hotep describes what Shu symbolizes:

> His long curved beard indicates that the ancient Egyptians or Kemetic people viewed him as a Netcher or force of nature. In the ancient Kemetic Scientific System of Cosmology, Shu represents the concept of the breath we breathe, which gives life to our physical bodies. It's also the atmosphere that surrounds the Earth and one of the four elements of creation, i.e., earth, air, fire and water.
>
> Egyptologists who studied ancient Egyptian civilization have known about this carving for thousands of years, yet no one ever equated Shu with Yoga. When we do a casual examination of his position and the symbols carved on the chair which includes the sun disk at the top of his head and two Cobra snakes, the connection with Yoga becomes obvious. The sun disk on top of his head corresponds to the crown chakra or energy center related to higher intelligence and enlightenment. The cobras correspond to two of the three main Nadis which according to Yogic science are channels through which energy or life force moves, nourishes and animates the human body.
>
> The position of Shu and all other myriad of Yoga positions we see represented in ancient Egyptian art and literature are not unique to that culture. You can find it in other parts of Africa and in the western hemisphere where Africans traveled thousands of years before Columbus."[3]

Hotep and other scholars provide strong evidence that connects yoga to an ancient African heritage. This opens the idea that there may be multiple cultural sources in different geographical locations that created their own yoga traditions of mindful-movement practices. We see this linkage of movement and spiritual connection in East Asian martial arts, and we see it in indigenous populations in North America with their traditions of drumming and dance. Ultimately, exploring the diverse origins of the practice only serves to further enrich the culture of yoga.

As teachers and practitioners of higher consciousness, we need to be open to the idea that yoga is much larger than we perceive it to be or have been taught to believe—and that its origins are likely far richer and more complex than what we think and understand about modern yoga culture today. It is important for black people and other people of color to know that their history is valid. The world belongs to them too, and their experiences and contributions matter. Black and brown lives matter and are an important part of the creation of the world we have today. People need to recognize this. Allowing a culture to know its roots, to take pride in its contribution to society, and to acknowledge its heritage and traditions takes nothing away from the dominant culture. It does not oppress the dominant culture, but rather, it enriches the experience of all of us. If people of color are celebrated for their accomplishments and are seen as equals in this culture, we can begin to dismantle white supremacy and finally focus on healing this society and this world.

YOGA IN SOUTH ASIA

As we've mentioned, the yoga many of us practice today is a combination of physical and spiritual practices from around the world, including Asia, Africa, and the West.

Though yoga in India dates back thousands of years, one of the biggest influences on modern yoga is from the lineage and teachings of Swami Vivekananda, an Indian Hindu monk born Narendranath Datta. He introduced the Indian philosophies of Vedanta and Yoga to the West in the late 1800s.[4] Tirumalai Krishnamacharya was another great Indian scholar and yoga master who studied in Tibet and was influential in the twentieth century. He blended hatha yoga techniques with calisthenics, gymnastics, and wrestling. Many students—B. K. S. Iyengar, K. Pattabhi Jois, Indra Devi, and T. K. V. Desikachar—adapted his techniques and became extremely influential in the postural yoga now practiced in much of the world. Many of today's most well-known teachers have practice lineages that connect them to this tradition.[5]

IMPORTANT YOGIC TEXTS THROUGHOUT HISTORY

Nothing in the world is static, and our knowledge about the history of yoga continues to grow and evolve. This section offers a brief look at the history and evolution of yoga by looking at some of its most important books—books that you may often hear your teacher reference in yoga class.

The Vedas

The Rig Veda—the Sanskrit word *rig* means "praise," and *veda* means "knowledge"— contains one of the first known written references to yoga. It is also one of the oldest known texts in any Indo-European language. Research suggests that at least some of its 1,028 hymns were composed in the third or even fourth millennium B.C.E. The Gayatri mantra, which is still chanted or played in the background in many modern classes, is found in the Rig Veda (3.62.10).

The other three Vedic hymn texts are the Yajur Veda ("Knowledge of Sacrifice"), Sama Veda ("Knowledge of Chants"), and Atharva Veda ("Knowledge of Atharvan," who was a famous fire priest).

The Bhagavad Gita

The Bhagavad Gita ("Lord's Song" in Sanskrit) is considered a valuable yoga scripture by many. It contains over seven hundred verses that encourage the reader to stand up against evil through a central message of action; to be alive is to be active and to move beyond our own egos to avoid the difficulties that life brings to us. Evidence suggests that the Bhagavad Gita was written around 500 B.C.E. It is embedded in the Mahabharata—one of the great national epics of India (another being the Ramayana).

The *Yoga Sutras* of Patanjali

No one knows much about the actual life of Patanjali, the author (or authors) of the *Yoga Sutras*, but this text is considered central to yoga practice by many teachers and students.

Scholars date the *Yoga Sutras* to around the fourth century B.C.E. This text comprises 196 (or 195 in some translations) aphorisms on yoga. It's interesting to note that only three of these sutras (2.46–2.48) even mention asana, and in those cases, it is likely referring to a seated posture for meditation, not the great variety of poses we see in classes today. The *Yoga Sutras* are divided into four chapters, or *padas*. The second chapter, "Sadhana Pada," focuses on practice (*sadhana* means practice) and is where you'll find the eight limbs of yoga, an eightfold path to liberation:

1. YAMA *Restraints, Moral Disciplines, or Vows*

Yama is the first limb and refers to disciplines or practices that give us direction on how to interact with the world around us. There are five yamas: *ahimsa* (nonviolence), *satya* (truthfulness), *asteya* (non-stealing), *brahmacharya* (right use of energy), and *aparigraha* (non-greed or non-hoarding).

2. NIYAMA *Observances*

The second limb, niyama, relates to our personal character and the ways we can improve our outlook on the world. There are also five niyamas, and they are intended to help move us closer to enlightenment through observation and action. The five niyamas are *saucha* (cleanliness), *santosha* (contentment), *tapas* (discipline or burning desire or, conversely, burning of desire), *svadhyaya* (self-study or self-reflection, and study of spiritual texts), and *ishvarapranidhana* (surrender to a higher power).

3. ASANA *Posture*

The word *asana* literally means "seat" in Sanskrit. Here, it is not referring to the ability to do the perfect wheel pose or a complicated arm balance. It is the opportunity to take a seat in meditation and witness your own life. Patanjali gives the instruction for asana as *sthira sukham asanam*: "the posture should be steady and easeful."

4. PRANAYAMA *Breathwork and Technique*

The word *prana* refers to "energy" or "life force." It is the essence or the energy that keeps us alive. *Pranayama* can be defined as "breath work," that is, breathing practices and techniques that can help us calm the mind and connect us more fully with the present moment. It can also be used as a way to connect with our bodies and reduce stress.

5. PRATYAHARA *Withdrawal of the Senses*

The word *pratya* means to "withdraw," "draw in," or "draw back," and *ahara* refers to anything we "take in" such as ideas, things we touch, sights, sounds, and smells. The practice of pratyahara is about being focused and aware of distractions that may pull us from meditation. The idea is to be present to the moment at hand, so that things like sensations and sounds don't easily distract the mind.

6. DHARANA *Focused Concentration*

The term *dhar* means "holding" or "maintaining," and *ana* means "other" or "something else." Dharana and pratyahara are connected. In order to intently focus on something, the senses must be withdrawn so that all attention is put on that one point of concentration.

7. DHYANA *Meditative Absorption*

We achieve *dhyana* is when we become fully engaged in our meditation without distraction. It is the actual state of meditation.

8. SAMADHI *Enlightenment*

The word *samadhi* comes from *sama*, meaning "same" or "equal," and *dhi*, meaning "to see." Samadhi is the ability to "see equally" or "truthfully," to become fully aware of the world around us, to make peace, and to have a clearer understanding of everything we come to learn through the eight limbs.

The *Hatha Yoga Pradipika*

This text's name means "light on hatha yoga." *Hatha* translates to "forceful," though "sun and moon"—referring to pairs of opposites—is also a popular translation. Very generally speaking "hatha yoga" is used to refer to the physical practices of yoga. The *Pradipika* dates back to the fifteenth century C.E. and is attributed to an author called Svatmarama. It discusses asana (here, referring to specific poses), pranayama, *shatkriya* (what could be described as "cleansing techniques"), and samadhi. The asana section describes fifteen poses and their purported benefits. Though they are primarily seated poses, for the most part, they are familiar to contemporary practitioners (in fact we include some of them in this book).

YOGA IN THE TWENTIETH CENTURY

Many yoga scholars see the beginning of modern yoga as occurring when Swami Vivekananda addressed the American public at the World Parliament of Religions in Chicago in 1893, receiving a standing ovation. While yoga teachers had come to the West prior to his visit, Swami Vivekananda made the most immediate and lasting impact. He was encouraged by his teacher Ramakrishna to share the teachings of yoga overseas, and his knowledge of yoga had a deep effect on many people. As he traveled throughout North America, he began attracting many new students to the power of yoga.

Another prominent yogi who helped popularize yoga in the West was Paramahansa Yogananda, who arrived in Boston in 1920. Paramahansa Yogananda was the creator of the Self-Realization Fellowship and author of the well-known book *The Autobiography of a Yogi*, which is still widely read today.

Both Swami Vivekananda and Paramahansa Yogananda presented a version of yoga that Western culture could understand, firmly rooted in self-improvement and spiritual enlightenment. In India, prior to yoga's migration to the West, hatha yoga (the physical practice) was often viewed as something utilized to make money by street performers or as the highly ritualized practices of members of secret sects. However, as yoga began to generate interest in the West as a physical and spiritual practice, the perception of hatha yoga started to shift within Indian and Hindu culture as well.

Yoga continued to gain more popularity in the West during the 1920s. A notable Yogi named Shri Yogendra arrived in Long Island in 1919 and captivated Americans with the power and strength of hatha yoga. Westerners loved the physicality of his version of this spiritual practice, and Shri Yogendra founded the American branch of Kaivalyadhama, an Indian organization created by the late Swami Kuvalayananda. Over the decades, this organization has contributed significantly to the scientific study of yoga.

Throughout the twentieth century, yoga continued to evolve from its diverse origins as a spiritual practice into a more physical, yet still mindful movement experience through the influence of many teachers—one of the most well known being Tirumalai Krishnamacharya. Often called "the father of modern yoga," Krishnamacharya cultivated *vinyasa* yoga—one of the most popular forms of yoga practice today. Vinyasa yoga combines breathing with movement and emphasizes the importance of teaching only what is appropriate for individual students. Many modern yoga classes focus on vinyasa-style movements that help students connect to joyful physical activity, similar to dance or calisthenics.

It is worth noting that many of the Indian yogis who had the most prominence in Western yoga culture had received a Western education. It is also worth noting that almost all of the influential teachers we have mentioned in this chapter have been cisgender men. This does not mean that people of other genders and those without Western educational backgrounds did not practice yoga or have great teachings to share. It is instead a reflection of societal norms and values. It is also important to mention that the history of yoga is not without scandal or harm. For example, during the time that we were writing this book, accounts of Ashtanga yoga founder Pattabhi Jois sexually assaulting students have been made public. Though a full discussion is beyond the scope of this book, we feel it is important for readers to be made aware of this, and for yoga teachers and students to learn more about how they can create safety in their classes, support survivors of sexual violence, and hold perpetrators accountable, no matter how "famous" or "authoritative" they may be. When looking back on history, it's important to ask ourselves, *Who's left out? Whose stories are not being told, and why?* And then to also ask ourselves, *Who's being left out of the conversation today? And what can we do to change things?*

YOGA TODAY

In the West, yoga has historically focused on individual practice for personal physical and spiritual development, but today the focus is changing again. Our perception of yoga is evolving from a physical practice aimed at self-fulfillment to a tool for fighting oppression and shaping consciousness. *Yoga* means unity, and unity means all of us, so it stands to reason that this was always the path of yoga—to fight injustice, to create peace, and to heal the world. We are beginning to understand how yoga can be a tool for the liberation of the mind, body, spirit, and soul on a much grander scale. Yoga is a tool for shaping critical consciousness. Yoga teaches the idea of a divine source that resides in all of us. That there is a light in all of us. At the root of who we are, we know that the injustices of the world must stop. The question is: How do we take action?

Having a spiritual or self-reflection practice, such as yoga, can help us see some of the most pressing questions of our day in a new way. For example, the social construct of race. We have many different species of flowers. We don't discriminate against daisies for not being roses. We see the beauty in both of these flowers. We see the beauty in the diversity of nature. Why is this so different for humankind? Why do we still allow racism, sexism, and other forms of discrimination against our neighbors? Why do we see the world suffering around us and allow it to continue? How can we use the practice of yoga to alleviate some of our suffering and to create equality?

The practice of yoga can broaden our scope of understanding and help us come to terms with the idea that we are a part of a larger consciousness, energy, or being. Once we share this understanding, then, and only then, can we abolish the systems that are unfair and unjust in the world.

Yoga can be an instrument for global change. Organizations such as Amplify and Activate, Yoga Service Council, Skill in Action, Accessible Yoga, Mind Body Solutions, Sanctuary in the City, and the Yoga and Body Image Coalition encourage using activism, self-reflection, and the spiritual teachings of yoga to change the world. These organizations shine a light on inequality and help teach us how to create a space for understanding. They make their work accessible through in-person events, social media, and online courses. Justice is compassion, equity, and universal love out loud. Yoga creates the idea that we are together in this struggle. The key is to bring more awareness to the collective struggle.

People are beginning to realize that the power for change comes from within. In our current state of consciousness, we believe in what yoga philosophy refers to as *asmita*, often translated as "ego." We often believe we are the masters of all we survey. We have become selfish and unaware of the world around us. We have forgotten that our actions and words have an impact on the lives of others. More important, we've forgotten that inaction and apathy are the destroyers of justice. As the great activist Martin Luther King Jr. tells us, "We may have all come on different ships, but we're in the same boat now."

In the human body, no one organ or limb can live separate from the entire system. All parts of the body must work together for it to function. The heart cannot work independently from the lungs and the stomach cannot work independently of the rest of the digestive system. The same can be said for the human condition. We often forget that we are all working together for a common goal of happiness, love, and fulfillment in this world. We must realize that we are all in this together, and we are hurting humanity with bigotry, exclusion, and hate. We must make room for change. As long as we maintain "us against them" mentalities, change will never happen. We cannot be truly free as a people, a society, or a culture if we do not allow *all* people to be free. To fully embrace the practice of yoga we must remember its meaning—union—and we must honor its rich and complex history.

2

Yoga, Accessibility, and Body Image

The body is political. Our bodies are the only vehicles we have in which to access the world. The way our bodies look often determines the type of treatment we receive or the access we have. In Western culture, able bodies, white bodies, and thin bodies have more access to resources than bodies that don't share those same characteristics. Bodies that are considered conventionally attractive have something called "beauty currency."

Regardless of your gender, looking the way that society deems "beautiful" opens many doors and provides greater access to resources. Not all of us receive the same access to justice, equity, and resources such as healthcare and the distribution of wealth. Our bodies come at a price. In a white-dominated culture, people of color are forced to continually prove their worth. Individuals on the fringe of what is considered conventionally beautiful must fight to be recognized for their humanity, experiences, and expertise. Skin color, disability, age, and size all factor heavily into how society perceives each of us.

Self-doubt is largely a by-product of cultural conditioning. For people of color and people who don't conform to societal and cultural norms, feelings of self-doubt and inadequacy become internalized. These messages of inferiority that we begin to feed ourselves are called "internalized oppression." Mainstream culture lays out the guide-lines of what is "normal" or what is "desirable," and this keeps marginalized groups from rising to our real potential. There are structural barriers in place that keep certain populations at a disadvantage. When we look at North America today, we can no longer dismiss structural racism, sexism, ageism, ableism, fat phobia, homophobia, and transphobia. Depending on the body you are in, your access to a safe and successful life may be in jeopardy. Why do the differences between our bodies create a divide?

> **DIANNE:** Speaking from my own experience, my fat black body comes with its own set of challenges. As a woman of color, my body is highly politicized and criticized. My skin tone and the length and texture of my hair play a major role in how I am perceived in the world. The darker I am, the less desirable, educated, or conventionally beautiful I am perceived to be, and the less bankable or salable power I have in the world. I once had a boss tell me he found me attractive because my features seemed more Caucasian. I quit my job the next day. Society has tried to tell me that my body is worth less than those of my white counterparts. Globally, this idea is reinforced. I don't receive the same access to justice or health care as my white counterparts. Police brutality toward brown and black bodies often doesn't receive adequate acknowledgment or punishment, as we have seen in the cases of Trayvon Martin, Eric Garner, and Sandra Bland. Women of color, particularly black women, are more likely to die in childbirth no matter their education or socioeconomic background, as documented by research at Harvard[6] and illustrated by the near-death experience of Serena Williams after the birth of her daughter.

Some questions for self-reflection and self-study to help us better define our humanity are: Why are white bodies considered to be worth more than nonwhite bodies, white male bodies worth more than female bodies, thin bodies worth more than fat bodies? Why are able bodies worth more than bodies with disabilities? Why are conforming bodies worth more than nonconforming bodies? These are the questions that can help us to better understand our humanity. These dichotomies create an "us versus them" paradigm. What, and who, do these polarities serve?

It would be nice to believe that all bodies are deemed intrinsically equal in our society, but it is simply not the case. We believe that all bodies are beautiful. All bodies are worthy. All bodies deserve our love, and respect, and care, regardless of their color, size, ability, or gender. We must begin to release our attachment to our cultural definitions of beauty and perfection, and we must begin to cherish and celebrate all of our bodies as they are.

The yogic principle of *ahimsa* or "non-harming" can inspire us to stop our hatred toward different bodies—including our own. Our hostility toward ourselves also creates hostilities toward each other. Our attachment to our ego and defining who we are in terms of the dominant paradigms of society and culture can keep us from exploring our true bias and prejudices.

Negative body image directly affects how we show up in the world. If we are consumed in our own self-hate, we cannot look at the world at large. We cannot advocate for ourselves or others when we are too busy hating on our bodies. The capitalist world banks on this inner conflict. It fuels our dissatisfaction under the guise of self-improvement: do better, be better, and buy this to help you do it.

But the inverse is also true: accepting ourselves helps us be better at accepting others. Positive body image also directly affects how we show up in the world. We do not need to buy into beauty standards that feed consumerism. We can celebrate our own beauty and the beauty of the lives that surround us.

BODY IMAGE

The term *body image* refers to the way we perceive our own bodies and the way we assume other people perceive us. Body image is a collection of ideas based on how we see ourselves in relationship to the outside world. Do we see ourselves as attractive, feminine, masculine, nonbinary, able-bodied, in bodies with disabilities, in older bodies, in younger bodies, in large bodies, or in small bodies? Our body image is influenced by messaging from friends, family, religion, culture, media, and society. Body image generally isn't based in fact and can be either positive or negative.

In the second chapter of the *Yoga Sutras* (2:35), we are taught that settling the mind allows for hostilities to cease. We begin by ceasing hostilities toward ourselves, and then begin ceasing hostilities toward others as well. When we allow our mind to settle, we begin to disengage from the cycle of insecurities that are borne into our conscious and subconscious lives. As we learn to release our attachments to the belief that our self-worth is skin deep, we begin to recognize that our attachments to the conventional are unnecessary.

Body image is largely a product of learned conditioning. Here are some facts about body image:

» Keeping people focused on body dissatisfaction through marketing helps the cosmetic and diet industries stay profitable. By presenting a physical ideal that is difficult to both achieve and maintain, these industries are assured continual growth and profits. As noted on the *Market Research* blog, "The total US weight loss market grew at an estimated 4.1% in 2018, from $69.8 billion to $72.7 billion. The total market is forecast to grow 2.6% annually through 2023."[7]

» Washington State University found that the average size of the American woman now falls between a 16 and an 18, the lower end of plus sizes.[8] The average size of a fashion model is 0–4.[9]

» The thin ideal is unachievable for most women and is likely to lead to feelings of self-devaluation, dysphoria (depression), and helplessness.[10]

» As Mario Palmer noted, "Approximately 91% of women are unhappy with their bodies and resort to dieting to achieve their ideal body shape. Unfortunately, only 5% of women naturally possess the body type often portrayed by Americans in the media."[11]

» "In a survey, more than 40% of women and about 20% of men agreed they would consider cosmetic surgery in the future. The statistics remain relatively constant across gender, age, marital status, and race."[12]

» "Students, especially women, who consume more mainstream media, place a greater importance on sexiness and overall appearance than those who do not consume as much."[13]

BODY IMAGE IN YOGA

In much of the contemporary practice of yoga, diet and fitness culture cross over. Most popular yoga teachers are thin, young, able-bodied, and white. Those are the gurus and experts that are lifted to celebrity status. Why is this so? Is it because they reflect the beauty, diet, and fitness culture ideal, which we have been conditioned to accept as normal and desirable? Asking questions about why we revere a yoga teacher can be a powerful tool for both self-reflection and cultural reflection.

At its root, the asana (or physical) yoga practice is designed to promote holistic wellness, as we aim to cultivate the mind-body connection. A healthy and regular yoga practice should be viewed as a self-care practice—a safe and comfortable tool for compassionate self-study. In this view of yoga, it is impossible to ignore a direct correlation between practicing yoga and the development of one's own body image.

Taking a closer look at the effects of yoga on body image should be a priority for everyone who practices yoga—especially teachers, both seasoned and aspiring, and people who work in yoga media. Teachers and yoga media can have a powerful impact on students' body image—either supporting a positive view of their self-worth or reinforcing a negative body image. It is important for teachers and professionals to look at the language we use in speaking about ourselves and how we project that on to others.

For years, mainstream yoga publications, websites, and clothing companies have carefully crafted a very specific image of what yoga looks like. Pictures of thin, almost exclusively white women are disproportionately featured in the advertising and promotion of yoga. Very rarely do we see an "average" or "regular" sized person doing a simple yoga pose. Even more rarely do we see someone with a disability, men, nonbinary people, older students, or other elements of diversity.

Thin, attractive, flexible, fair-skinned women sell yoga magazines. This aesthetic was very carefully crafted as aspirational marketing. Society creates this image so that corporations can continue making money off our insecurities about ourselves and our bodies.

The notion that a "yoga body" must be young, thin, and flexible illustrates how pervasive the ideals of beauty are in our perceptions of yoga practice. Many yoga teachers come to this practice with natural flexibility and the privilege of an able body. Sometimes, however, this privilege may inadvertently affect our ability to serve students with body types that are different than our own. Due to a lack of understanding, we may feel unsure of how to modify poses for students who come to our classes with different body types and levels of ability. Yet students come to us for guidance when they are unsure how to serve themselves or adapt the practice to their bodies.

While it is not our intention to exclude students because of our own lack of understanding or unfamiliarity, it happens! When we neglect to provide an atmosphere of understanding and appreciation for different body types and abilities in our classes, we can cause students to feel marginalized and alienated from the asana practice. In this way, we can leave students feeling as though they are unable to execute or experiment with a particular posture, or worse, we can leave them feeling as though the entire asana practice and all its benefits are beyond their reach. Sadly, this then creates the internal message that there is something "wrong" with the student's body, and thus perpetuates negative impressions, thoughts, feelings, and opinions.

We firmly believe that all bodies are yoga bodies.

In actuality, it is not the student's body that needs adjusting in a pose, but rather the asana or posture itself that requires an adjustment or the use of a different prop for support. By adapting the posture to the student's body, as opposed to shaping the student's body into the posture, we as teachers can provide an atmosphere of understanding and appreciation for all bodies within our classes. As a result, we can come to serve all of our students in an effort to improve and elevate a positive and healthy lifestyle, regardless of a student's body size or ability.

We can apply this same understanding of all bodies as yoga bodies in our own personal practice as well. The words we use to talk to ourselves have power. We don't need to believe that we must change ourselves to fit a pose or a class or a perception of a yoga lifestyle. Instead, we can adjust a pose or a class or a lifestyle to fit us right where we are. We can meet and celebrate our own unique bodies and experiences, and we can customize our yoga practice to benefit our unique bodies, minds, and spirits.

APPRECIATING OUR BODIES

The most important step in appreciating our bodies is to meet ourselves where we are.

As yoga teachers, we can create a truly inclusive yoga class by coming to understand and appreciate different body types and abilities and by learning how to adapt a pose and a practice to fit different kinds of bodies. We can share inspiration from, and promote the work of, a diverse range of teachers. We can focus on encouraging students to come to the mat and accepting where they are in their own practice. We can recognize that some students come to the mat with a genetic privilege, and we can celebrate that all bodies are yoga bodies.

Many of these ideas also apply to our personal practice. We can work on identifying the stories we tell ourselves about our worth, power, or beauty—on and off the mat. We can begin to question the negative stories, and we can begin to celebrate where we are in our lives and in our practice, regardless of how it looks. We can look for teachers and media that highlight accessibility and acceptance. We can focus on coming to the mat for any amount of time, and we can know that we don't need to change to find benefit.

The Health at Every Size (HAES) movement makes the powerful claim that we can be healthy people regardless of how our bodies look. Their website (www.haes community.com) is a wonderful resource for learning about how to respect every body, challenge our assumptions, find compassionate self-care practices, and work for justice. Other groups, such as the Yoga and Body Image Coalition, are active in trying to change the dominant narrative around yoga and health, and they also offer excellent resources.

We don't need to overcome our bodies—we need to overcome our attachment. What if we could overcome our attachment to diet culture, the beauty industry, and celebrity culture? What might we be capable of if we began to view our bodies with satisfaction instead of distrust?

At its core, attachment is based on fear and insecurity. When you forget your true Self—which the yoga tradition tells us is pure consciousness, pure potentiality—you begin to believe that you need something outside of yourself in order to achieve happiness.

And yet, you don't. You are worthy just as you are.

This book offers ideas for how to adapt poses to all kinds of bodies, so you can customize your practice or support your students. It also offers supportive language in talking about poses and bodies—this can shape how your talk to yourself or to your students. We hope this book can serve as a tool to help you begin to accept all bodies—your own and others.

You might consider these questions on your journey:

» The first step in accepting our bodies is letting go of our attachment to beauty and perfection as defined by our culture. What if we saw all bodies as equal regardless of color, size, and gender?

» Do we see yoga as an individual pursuit or as something that fosters connection to each other?

» Can we start to integrate our own yoga and mindfulness practices with the collective work of social justice?

» In our self-study, can we recognize our own bias and explore how it affects our lives and the world around us?

» How do we engage with others who are different from us?

» If we see yoga as unity, how can we serve our communities—either through working with local organizations or with larger groups like the Yoga Service Council?

3

Yoga Practice Basics

Hey, beginners, this chapter is especially for you! These are our top ten tips for getting started with yoga.

Teachers and seasoned yogis, you can share these tips the next time someone says "I want to try yoga; how do I start?"

1. GATHER YOUR BASIC SUPPLIES

You don't need to spend a ton of money on fancy swag to start your practice—in fact, no one *ever* needs to spend a ton of money on fancy yoga swag. That's part of what makes yoga such an accessible activity: it doesn't require much space or equipment, and you can start your practice right at home. However, there are a few things you may want to have on hand before you begin:

» **COMFORTABLE CLOTHING:** We're not talking $200 yoga pants; just something you can move around in without restriction (we even practice at home in our stretchy jeans sometimes so we can squeeze in a few minutes of yoga as time allows). You might also want to avoid shirts that are too baggy or "flowy" because they have a tendency to fly up in your face in upside-down poses like downward-facing dog, making it difficult to see where you're going and what your legs and feet are doing. If you're a person with breasts, you'll want to have a supportive sports bra. And while lots of yogis practice barefoot, if you're not a barefoot kind of person, we recommend getting some socks that grip to keep you from slipping (search for "barre socks" online and you'll find plenty of options). For some people, finding some special yoga clothes that they like and feel comfortable in can be extra motivation for practice.

» **A MAT:** Okay, this might sound almost blasphemous, but you don't *need* a mat to practice yoga! However, you may be required to use one if you're practicing at a studio or gym (many have mats that you can borrow or rent), and often, practicing on a mat at home can be more comfortable than practicing on carpet or bare floor. While yoga mats can be expensive, there are many affordable options, both in stores and online.

» **ANY PROPS YOU MIGHT FIND HELPFUL:** If you're practicing in a studio or gym, they will likely have props available for you to use. If you're practicing at home, you may find it useful to have a few basic props on hand. Chapter 5 covers some common yoga props, and there you'll find suggestions for household items you can use as substitutes.

2. FIND A BEGINNER-FRIENDLY CLASS OR VIDEO PRACTICE TO DO AT HOME

It's important for students and teachers to remember that "beginner" doesn't necessarily mean "easy." A beginner is simply someone who is new to yoga, and one beginner's goals and needs may vary widely from the next. Also keep in mind that there are *many* different kinds of yoga out there. If you try a class and you don't like it, that doesn't necessarily mean you don't like or won't like yoga at all, just that that wasn't the class for you. Here are some tips for finding a class that's a good fit:

» If you're planning to try out a studio or gym, give them a call or shoot them an email and let them know you're a beginner along with what you're looking for from a yoga class (something relaxing or something physically challenging, for example).

» If you're working with an injury or specific physical limitations, look for classes labeled "accessible yoga" or "adaptive yoga." "Chair yoga" may also be a good fit. Keep in mind that some chair yoga classes are done entirely seated, whereas others involve standing and/or lying or sitting on the floor using a chair as a prop or balance support. If you're trying an in-person chair yoga class, it's a good idea to ask ahead of time if the class is all-seated or not if you have a need or preference one way or the other. If you're practicing online, search for "all seated" or "completely seated" chair yoga if needed or desired.

» If you're looking for something relaxing and slower-paced, look for *gentle* or *restorative yoga* classes, most of which tend to be beginner-friendly. Yin yoga (see next point) is also slower-paced and more on the meditative side, though not all classes are appropriate for all beginners, so look for a "Yin for Beginners" class online, or let the studio/teacher know that you're a beginner before trying an in-person class.

» If you want to increase flexibility/mobility try a Yin yoga class, which involves holding (primarily seated or lying) poses for a set time (usually a few minutes per pose) and working toward your "edge"—the place where you feel a sensation of stretch, but not one that's so extreme or uncomfortable that you're in pain or can't breathe with ease. You might also try a class that blends yoga and myofascial release (MFR), which involves using tools like massage balls and foam rollers for self-massage.

» If you're looking to add yoga as a means of cross-training or recovery for an athletic endeavor, look for a class geared toward your particular sport or activity (for example, "yoga for runners" or "yoga for cyclists"). Often, these classes are geared toward athletes who are also yoga newbies. Keep in mind that some of these classes will be more "recovery-focused," putting more emphasis on stretching, myofascial-release practices, and relaxation, while others will be more focused on helping you to enhance particular skills (such as endurance), and still others will focus more on cross-training: working areas of the body that your sport or activity may neglect. Depending on your needs and goals, inquire with the studio or teacher about what to expect, or read the class description so you know what to expect from an online class.

» If you're looking for a class that's physically challenging and/or more fast-paced, try *vinyasa yoga* or *power yoga*. At a studio, you might look for "all levels" classes, which often welcome beginners (though be sure to let them know that you're new, so the teacher knows to explain any "yoga jargon" ahead of time). Some studios also offer "vinyasa 101" classes for beginners. Online, look for a beginner or level-1 class. If you really want a *workout* try a *HIIT yoga* class (high intensity interval training). These classes typically involve movements that are simple but nonetheless physically challenging, with push-ups, burpees, and jump squats interspersed with yoga poses.

» If you want a class that's focused on breaking down poses step-by-step, look for the term *alignment-based* or try a style like Iyengar yoga, which is known for being very alignment-focused. Most Iyengar yoga studios offer beginner-specific classes, and you can also find Iyengar classes for beginners online.

» If you're not sure what you want, and you just want to try some yoga already, an in-person or online class labeled "yoga for beginners" is a good starting place. From there, you can figure out what you like, what you don't, and make your search a little more refined moving forward.

For more information about online classes we teach or recommend, see the Recommended Resources section.

3. FIND A DURATION THAT FITS YOUR SCHEDULE AND NEEDS

Want to know one of yoga's best-kept secrets? It doesn't have to take a long time! Sure, you'll find some people who say a yoga class "really should be ninety minutes," but frankly, we disagree. Doing yoga regularly, or even just at all is *way* more important than doing it for a long time. And really, you're more likely to benefit from a little bit of yoga done each day (or most days) than a lot of yoga done once in a blue moon. If you're short on time, online classes can be particularly beneficial because along with longer classes, you can find lots of classes in a variety of styles that range from ten to forty-five minutes each. While yoga-studio classes are traditionally on the longer side, more and more studios and gyms are offering sixty- and even forty-five-minute-class options. And many offer "lunch break" classes that are on the shorter side so that you can truly fit yoga into a work break and still have time to get to and from class. Starting small is a great way to make yoga a habit that sticks!

4. CARVE OUT YOUR YOGA SPACE

Creating a dedicated spot for practice at home can encourage you to return to your mat regularly. Keep your mat there along with any props you have so that you can easily "stop, drop, and yoga" anytime you need to. This spot could be right next to your bed, in a corner in the living room, or anywhere you have a mat-sized bit of space. If possible, it's helpful to set up your yoga space so that you don't have to move furniture around. That way there's one less obstacle between you and your yoga!

5. MAKE A YOGA DATE WITH YOURSELF

Put your yoga time in your calendar, set an alarm, and make your "me time" nonnegotiable. Remember, it doesn't have to take a long time, and a little bit can go a long way. Decide, for example, that you're going to do a fifteen-minute yoga class at 7:00 a.m., Monday, Wednesday, and Friday. Put this info in your phone calendar (and maybe even add a link to the class for easy access!) or write it down. Choose a time that's realistic for you: If you're not a morning person, go on a yoga-lunch date with yourself, or practice in the evening. The best time for yoga is the time that you're actually going to do yoga!

6. RECRUIT A FRIEND!

Starting a new activity can be more fun and less overwhelming if you don't go it alone. If you don't know anyone personally who's interested in doing yoga with you, check out yoga-related Facebook groups, and other online forums to connect with other beginners. These can also be great sources of support and helpful places to ask questions. Do a little searching and find a group that jibes with you and your goals.

7. FIND YOUR GO-TO SEQUENCE

Whether it's an online class or one of the sequences in this book (chapter 17 includes lots of options), find a short yoga sequence that you enjoy and make it your go-to. That way when you unroll your mat at home, you don't have to figure out what to do—you already know and you can dive right in!

8. SET A GOAL

Setting a yoga-related goal is a great way to begin and maintain your practice. While you could make your goal about learning a particular pose, we recommend starting with something that's easier to track: for example, "practice yoga for at least ten minutes every day for a month" or "attend three yoga classes this week." When creating a goal, make it SMART—specific, measurable, attainable, relevant, and time-bound. Avoid something super vague like "start practicing yoga" (instead, "practice yoga for fifteen minutes before work, M–F" would be more clear); make it something that's easy to assess (either you practiced on those days or you didn't); make sure it's something you can actually do (don't resolve to practice every day at 3:00 a.m. for an hour, for example, unless you're *really* sure that's something you can do); make it relevant to your interests (hopefully you're practicing yoga because you want to); and set a time limit (resolve to practice for your set amount of time—a month or a week, for example, instead of making it a "forever" thing). At the end of your designated time frame, see what worked and what didn't, if you'd like to do a little more or a little less in the future, and set a brand new goal based upon what you learned.

9. BREATHE

Want to know another yoga secret? It's not just about the poses. Yoga means *union*, or *to yoke*, and anytime you're present with yourself, connecting your mind, body, and breath, you're practicing yoga. Take a moment to simply notice your breath: When you're breathing in, when you're breathing out. What places in your body move as you breathe? If possible, can you breathe in and out through your nose? (It's okay if you can't; breathe however you comfortably can.) Can you make your inhale and exhale the same length? Perhaps count your inhale and exhale (three counts in, three counts out, or shorter or longer depending on what feels natural to you). Can you do this for five breaths? Guess what? You're doing yoga!

10. MAKE IT FUN!

The best way to start something new and stick with it is to actually enjoy it! Remember that yoga isn't about doing anything perfectly. It's about getting to know yourself better, and, like in any relationship, fun is important. Let yourself be silly. Put on your favorite playlist to accompany your home practice, give yourself permission to laugh and even goof off a little. Dance around in between poses, make up your own fun poses, don't be afraid to mess up! (Here's another yoga secret: you can't actually "mess up" when you're doing yoga!)

4

Breath and Drishti

Breath work and *drishti* (a focal point for our gaze) are two elements of a yoga practice that can help us connect with our bodies and customize the practice for ourselves—whether in a class or at home. This chapter offers an overview to help you better understand what they are, how they shape our practice, and how we can choose to use them (or not).

YOGA AND THE BREATH

Often you'll hear people say that what differentiates yoga from other forms of movement is that "yoga is all about the breath." This isn't untrue (though there are other breath-centric forms of movement out there besides yoga—Pilates for one), but what does it mean exactly? What is the role of the breath in yoga?

The answer you get will depend on who you ask and the style of yoga they practice or teach. Different styles of yoga emphasize different aspects of the breath and employ different breathing techniques, but in general, all styles of yoga have this in common: *when you practice yoga, you pay attention to your breath*.

This is significant because breathing is a function of your autonomic nervous system, which means for the most part you don't have to think about it. While this is largely a *good* thing, there are some benefits to occasionally thinking about, and consciously influencing, the way that you breathe. For example, we can use the breath as a tool to help us de-stress, we can begin to notice the way in which our breathing habits relate to our emotions, we can use the breath to help us focus, and we can also use it to make our movements on the mat feel more easeful and seamless. Here, we'll explore some key breath-related terms you'll often come across in yoga classes and some common *pranayama* (breath work) exercises that you may wish to explore.

DIAPHRAGMATIC BREATHING

Generally speaking, we're always using our diaphragm to breathe. That's because the diaphragm is the muscle that moves our lungs. When we inhale, the diaphragm, which sits below the middle and lower ribs, contracts and moves downward, causing the lungs to expand and fill with air, and it relaxes on the exhale as we expel that air. You might say that the diaphragm is what "breathes" the lungs. So what does it mean when a yoga teacher says to "breathe diaphragmatically" or "breathe from your diaphragm"? (*Note to yoga teachers*: Please don't tell your students to "breathe into" their diaphragms. That's not really possible!)

When we're stressed out, and our sympathetic "fight or flight" nervous system is active, we tend to breathe more shallowly, which you may hear described as "chest breathing." This means that we're relying a little more on "accessory breathing muscles" (smaller muscles of the chest) to move our lungs. Consciously adjusting our breathing so that the accessory breathing muscles do less and the diaphragm, the "main muscle of breathing," does more can help take us out of fight or flight mode by activating our parasympathetic nervous system—the "rest and digest" nervous system. How? By stimulating an important nerve called the vagus nerve, which innervates the diaphragm and, when stimulated, signals the parasympathetic nervous system to "switch on." Kind of cool, right?

But how do we "breathe diaphragmatically" and get the "rest and digest" nervous system to activate? We aim to find a breath that's smooth, even, and full. Now, when you first start to observe your breath, it may not be particularly "smooth," it may feel kind of "jumpy," or "rough," which is normal and fine. The more you observe and work with your breath, the more it naturally will start to smooth out.

So just start by noticing: When are you breathing in, and when are you breathing out? Can you breathe in and out through your nose if possible? Can you find an inhale and exhale that are even in length and quality? This means that one is just as important as the other. And maybe you count: three counts in, three counts out, for example (or four, or five, or six—whatever feels natural and easeful). Then start noticing the places that move as you breathe. What's expanding? What's contracting? The answer will depend somewhat on the position of your body.

IF YOU'RE SITTING OR STANDING UPRIGHT, see if you can expand your ribcage on your inhale by breathing into the back and sides of your ribcage (maybe even place your hands there). You'll likely notice some movement in your upper abdomen too. Your lower abdomen will be relatively still, because your core muscles are engaging to keep you upright. As you exhale, see if you can keep some of that expansion and find a little more engagement in your belly, drawing it in slightly, as though you were cinching a drawstring between your two frontal hip bones. Can you keep some of that engagement on your next inhale as you expand the sides and back of your ribcage? Can you keep some of that expansion on your exhale as you reengage your low belly? And so on.

IF YOU'RE LYING DOWN ON YOUR BACK, you'll notice more expansion in your abdomen on your inhale. Simply allow it to move as it will. On your inhalation, as your diaphragm contracts and moves downward, it will push into the organs below, causing your belly to push outward (you're not literally breathing air into your belly, but your belly will move as you breathe). As you exhale and your diaphragm moves back up, your belly naturally draws in.

IF YOU'RE LYING ON YOUR BELLY, as in crocodile pose (see page 211) or doing a pose like child's pose where your belly is pressing into your thighs, the movement of your belly will be restricted by the floor or your legs underneath it, so you'll notice more movement in the back and sides of your ribcage, and maybe your lower back too.

These are just a few examples—it can be interesting to observe the effects that different yoga poses have on the movement of the breath!

You might notice that after spending a few moments observing your breath, working with your breath, that it naturally starts to smooth out.

In general, "diaphragmatic breathing" in yoga refers to breathing consciously, smoothly, and fully. It doesn't mean breathing as long or as deeply as you can, but rather noticing your breath, seeing if you can let go of any places where you may be holding, gripping, or restricting your breath, and simply allowing your breath to "move" however it wants to.

BREATHING THROUGH THE NOSE

In yoga, we're often instructed to breathe in and out through the nose, as opposed to (for example) Pilates, where we may be asked to breathe in through the nose and out through the mouth, or a more aerobic-type class like cycling or Zumba where we often *have* to breathe through our mouth in order to breathe at all! But why?

Okay, first things first: the important thing is that you're *breathing*. So if you have a cold or another reason why breathing in and out through your nose isn't really working for you, don't sweat it, just breathe.

Breathing through the nose has some benefits, like bringing more oxygen into the lower lobes of the lungs, which have more parasympathetic nerve receptors, further supporting diaphragmatic breathing, and releasing more nitric oxide, which allows our cells to get more oxygen. The nose also has a more efficient filtering system than the mouth.

In general, breathe through your nose if you comfortably can, but just make sure you're breathing!

A note to teachers: While offering helpful hints and suggestions for breath work is important, it's also crucial that we don't micromanage our students' breathing. It's very possible that people in our classes have experienced trauma, and while breath work can be a useful tool for working with trauma, what is or is not useful or appropriate can vary greatly from person to person. Not all breathing practices are appropriate for all people, and it's not our job to try to "heal" anyone's trauma—with breath work or any other practice—but rather to cultivate a safe, welcoming environment where we encourage all students to make the choices that are right for them.

UJJAYI BREATH

Particularly if you attend vinyasa yoga classes, you may be taught to practice *ujjayi* breath. *Ujjayi* literally means "victory," though this type of breathing is sometimes described as "ocean breath" or "Darth Vader breath" because of its audible quality.

Here's how you do it:

First, inhale through your nose as you normally would, then exhale through your mouth, as though you were fogging up a mirror. Do this a couple of times.

Then see if you can breathe in that same way, but keep your mouth closed on the exhale. When you breathe this way, you slightly engage the muscles in the back of your throat, creating a sound that's loud enough for you and maybe a person standing next to you to hear.

You can stick with ujjayi on just the exhale, or, see if you can engage these muscles to create a slight whisper sound on the inhale as well.

Keep your inhales and exhales smooth and even as you practice ujjayi breath.

Some people find that ujjayi provides a good focal point for their mind as they practice, helping them to remain present and aware.

COMMON PRANAYAMA PRACTICES

Prana is a Sanskrit term that means "life force." While prana is not the same thing as breath itself, according to the yoga tradition, it's the force that moves the breath, and that which animates all life. "Vital energy" is another common translation of *prana*. *Yama* is a Sanskrit word that means "control." Though *prana* isn't exactly synonymous with "breath," *pranayama* is often translated as "breath control" and refers to exercises and practices in which we work with the breath intentionally, in various ways—usually to cultivate a particular effect, like helping us to feel calm or energized.

Another way you can look at the word *pranayama* is to break it up into the words *prana* and *ayama* (in Sanskrit, when you combine a word that ends in *a* like *prana* with a word that begins with *a* like *ayama* you get rid of one of the *a*'s, so instead of *pranaayama* it's *pranayama*). *Ayama* means "non-control," so according to this definition, pranayama is less about controlling the breath, and more about letting the breath (or perhaps more accurately the vital force that moves the breath) do its thing. Some teachers and students prefer this definition because it's less strict/rigid and more about allowing than forcing.

However you choose to break down the etymology, in the context of yoga today *pranayama* is generally used to refer to breathing exercises. We'll look at a few of the most common ones.

NADI SHODHANA (ALTERNATE-NOSTRIL BREATHING)

Nadi shodhana is often one of the first pranayama practices that yoga students learn. It's generally taught at the beginning or end of a yoga class to cultivate a calming effect and is also a nice lead-in for meditation practice. You can incorporate it in your home practice in any of these ways.

Its name (which you may sometimes see written as *nadi shodhanam*) translates to "channel purification," and refers to the *nadis*, the subtle energy channels that the yoga tradition describes as residing within us. From a literal, physical sense, though, you're breathing through one nostril at a time.

There are many different ways to practice nadi shodhana—we'll explore a simple one.

- Begin sitting up tall, on the floor (perhaps on a blanket or bolster to be comfortable on the floor) or in a chair. You can close your eyes if you like.

- Take the index and middle finger of your dominant hand and curl them into your palm so that just your thumb, ring, and pinky finger are sticking out.

- Sit tall and bring your hand to your nose. If your right hand is your dominant hand, bring your right thumb to rest lightly outside your right nostril and your right ring finger to rest lightly outside your left nostril.

- If your left hand is your dominant hand, bring your left thumb to rest lightly outside your left nostril and your left ring finger to rest lightly outside of your right nostril.

- Inhale through both nostrils.

- Then, lightly block your left nostril and exhale through your right nostril.

- Lightly block your right nostril and inhale through your left.

- Do this three times total: exhale right, inhale left.

- Then, after your third inhale on the left, exhale through your left nostril.

- Then lightly block your left nostril and inhale through your right.

- Do this three times total: exhale left, inhale right.

- After your third inhale on the right, release your hand and exhale through both nostrils.

- Take three regular breaths (inhales and exhales) through both nostrils to complete your practice.

Keep in mind that this pattern (exhale right, inhale left three times, exhale left, inhale right three times) is one of many nadi shodhana patterns you may come across in yoga classes and trainings.

TIP If you can't or don't want to physically block one nostril, you can instead visualize air moving in and out through one nostril at a time for a similar and effective practice.

KAPALABHATI (SKULL-SHINING BREATH)

This breathing practice is often taught at the beginning of yoga classes, or before other pranayama practices and meditation in order to make breathing through the nose clearer and easier.

TIP Blow your nose before you do this one!

Kapalabhati means "skull shining," or "skull illuminating," perhaps referring to the clarity of mind and "brightness" that many practitioners feel after doing it. It involves a quick, forceful exhale followed by a passive inhale. It sometimes goes by the name "breath of fire." Like nadi shodhana, different yoga styles teach it in different ways. We'll explore one of those ways.

> Begin sitting tall, eyes closed if you like. Place one hand on your lower belly. As you do this practice, you'll try to keep the movement in your belly, while keeping your chest relatively still. Keeping a hand on your belly can help!

> Inhale and exhale through your nose as you normally would.

> Then, inhale to just half your capacity.

> Exhale forcefully through your nose, contracting your low belly and making a "sniffing" sound through your nose.

> Let your inhale arise naturally.

> Repeat.

> Start slowly (think one exhale per second) and do this eleven times total to start. Conclude with a powerful exhale, then inhale naturally and take a few easy resting breaths when you're done.

> Repeat this two more times if you like.

As you get comfortable with kapalabhati, you can speed it up and do more repetitions. Popular numbers include 27, 54, and 108. The number 108 is important in the yoga tradition (27 and 54 are multiples of 108). It often shows up in scripture and in traditional rituals and practices—to offer one example, a *mala*, the prayer beads used as a tool for meditation, typically has 108 beads.

Remember: Forceful exhales, passive inhales.

BHASTRIKA (BELLOWS BREATH)

Bhastrika, which means "bellows breath" (think of a bellows fanning the flames of a fireplace), is similar to kapalabhati, but it includes a forceful exhale *and* inhale. It's said to have a particularly energizing effect.

Here's how to do it:

Sit tall. Here too, you want the movement to be primarily in your belly, not your chest, so it can be helpful to place a hand on your lower belly.

Inhale and exhale through your nose as you normally would.

Then, inhale to just half your capacity.

Exhale forcefully through your nose, contracting your low belly and making a "sniffing" sound through your nose.

Immediately follow with a forceful inhale, also creating a sniffing sound.

Start slowly, aiming for one exhale/inhale per second and do eleven repetitions. Finish with a powerful exhale, then take a few resting breaths. Repeat two more times if you like.

As with kapalabhati, once you're comfortable with bhastrika, you can pick up the pace and add repetitions.

Remember: Powerful exhale *and* inhale.

FIND YOUR DRISHTI

In yoga, your *drishti* refers to your gaze or focal point. In Ashtanga yoga, there are nine very specific drishti points: the tip of the nose, between the eyebrows, the navel, the hand, the toes, far to the right, far to the left, the thumbs, and up to the sky. These specific drishtis correspond with specific poses (for example, in an Ashtanga class you may be asked to gaze at your navel in downward dog or to your toes in a seated forward bend).

In other styles of yoga, however (including the yoga that we both practice and teach) the concept of drishti is broader—it can refer to anywhere you gaze or look. Typically, we hear the term used in the context of tricky balance poses (such as one-legged standing poses) as a tool to help with balance. You may have heard a yoga teacher tell you to "find your drishti" in warrior III, for example. Really, though, gazing at a focal point could be useful in almost any pose to help you remain present and aware. "Find your drishti" doesn't necessarily mean "stare at whatever happens to be in front of you," though. It means to focus your gaze on the place that will best support your needs and goals for practice. For example, do you want to feel steadier and more grounded? Do you want to challenge your balance? Here are some helpful tips for finding your drishti in a standing balance posture:

» Choose a spot that's not too close to you (about six to ten feet in front of you is a pretty good guideline to start).

» Choose something that's not moving (i.e., not another person, because if they fall out of the pose, you might too!).

» A focal point that's closer to the ground can help you stay steadier. If you'd like to test your balance, on the other hand, you might choose something higher up.

5

How to Use Props

Props are wonderful tools to enhance your yoga practice—whether you are a beginner or an experienced practitioner. Some students (and teachers) may feel resistant to using a prop, worrying that it shows they are not capable of a pose or are deficient in some way. We believe the opposite to be true! Props can dramatically change your experience of a pose, can make something either more accessible or more challenging, and can help you make wise choices for your body just as it is. We don't see the use of props as a lesser modification, but rather a wonderful variation to help customize your practice.

Here are the props we use for many of the pose variations in this book along with suggestions for how to use them, where to find them, and common household items you can swap out instead. We also share some of the most common myths about working with props, followed by the truth!

YOGA BLOCKS

Also known as . . .

You'll sometimes hear these referred to as "yoga bricks."

Common uses

To "lengthen" your arms or legs, bringing the ground closer to or farther away from you; to squeeze or push into in order to activate specific muscles; to prop up body parts for added comfort; to give you a boost in arm balances and inversions.

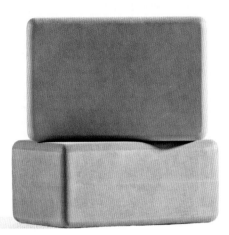

How they vary

Blocks can vary in material and thickness (ranging from around two to four inches thick in general). Foam blocks are lighter and often cheaper, though less environmentally friendly. Cork, wood, or bamboo blocks are often greener alternatives and they're also on the heavier/sturdier side.

Where to find them

Yoga blocks are ubiquitous these days! You can find them in athletic stores, department stores, maybe even your local supermarket, as well as lots of places online.

Easy substitutions

Many people recommend thick books as a block alternative, though it's important for yoga teachers to keep in mind that depending on a person's cultural background and/or religious beliefs, they may not be comfortable placing books on the floor. If you need something to place under your hands, sturdy water bottles, an upside-down (empty!) wastebasket, or a set of sturdy dumbbells can also be great block alternatives. If you're looking for something to squeeze or press into, a rubber ball (like a child's play ball) or folded blanket or towel can work great.

YOGA STRAP

Also known as . . .

A "yoga belt."

Common uses

To lasso a limb that you can't quite reach, to add resistance—to give you something to "pull apart" or "press out against."

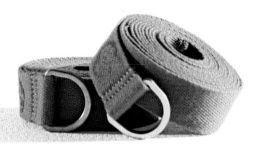

How they vary

Straps come in different lengths (often ranging from six to ten inches) and have different types of clasp (typically plastic buckles or metal "D rings"). We like longer straps because they're a bit more versatile in their use. Metal D rings are often a little easier to cinch than the plastic buckles, and they're more eco-friendly.

Where to find them

Straps are common props that you'll typically find in all the same places as blocks.

Easy substitutions

A bathrobe tie, a dog leash, a jump rope, an actual belt, a necktie, a long sock (if you just need a little bit of length).

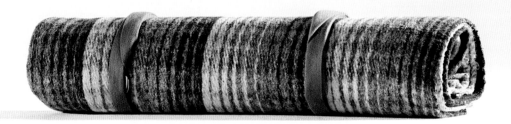

BLANKET

Common uses

To elevate a body part (like your seat or your heels), to add extra cushioning and support.

How they vary

Blankets come in different sizes, materials, and thickness. This is important to keep in mind if you're allergic to any material (such as wool) or need to fold a blanket in a particular way. Blankets sold on yoga websites, at yoga studios, and those labeled "saddle blankets" are typically easy to fold up for common yoga variations.

Where to find them

Online, at yoga studios, from local artisans, maybe even on your living room couch!

Easy substitutions

Large towels; any blanket, afghan, or thin sleeping bag you may have around the house; a rolled-up yoga mat is often a great substitute for a rolled-up blanket.

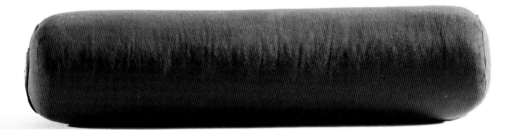

BOLSTER

Common uses

To fill in space, to add cushioning or support, to literally "bolster" you in almost any way you can imagine!

How they vary

Bolsters come in all different shapes, sizes, densities, and heights.

Where to find them

Yoga studios, online, some places that sell other yoga props (such as department and athletic supply stores).

Easy substitutions

Thick pillows or cushions, a thickly rolled blanket. You can also put together an especially thick, firm, and cozy makeshift bolster by rolling up a couple of blankets (or even rolling up a blanket or two around a thick, rolled-up yoga mat), and then using a couple of yoga straps or belts to hold them in place.

WALL

Common uses

To stand in front of or next to for support, to press into for feedback, to climb up, to hold you steady in an inversion.

Where to find them

Your home, your yoga studio, or any indoor space where you practice.

Easy substitutions

If you're practicing outside, a sturdy tree makes a lovely wall-ternative!

CHAIR

Common uses

To provide balance support, to "raise the floor" and/or elevate your hands or feet, to shift the symmetry of a pose in order to stretch and strengthen different muscle groups, to serve as a steady platform to begin to explore arm balancing. When practicing chair-supported variations, we recommend having all four chair legs on your mat in order to prevent the chair from sliding.

How they vary

You can buy special backless "yoga chairs" that can be more versatile to work with, but most of the time a simple folding chair or even your average kitchen chair will do.

Where to find them

You can find backless yoga chairs online (they're sometimes referred to as "Iyengar chairs"); regular folding chairs are available in multiple places online and in many department stores and superstores.

Easy substitutions

Most of the time any sturdy chair will work just fine for yoga. Depending on the pose variation, you may be able to sub a sofa, ottoman, coffee table, bed, or other piece of furniture as well.

ROLLED-UP YOGA MAT

Common uses

To place under your knees for support and/or press into to engage specific muscle groups, to elevate your toes or heels in order to make a pose more or less intense, to support your back heel in standing poses.

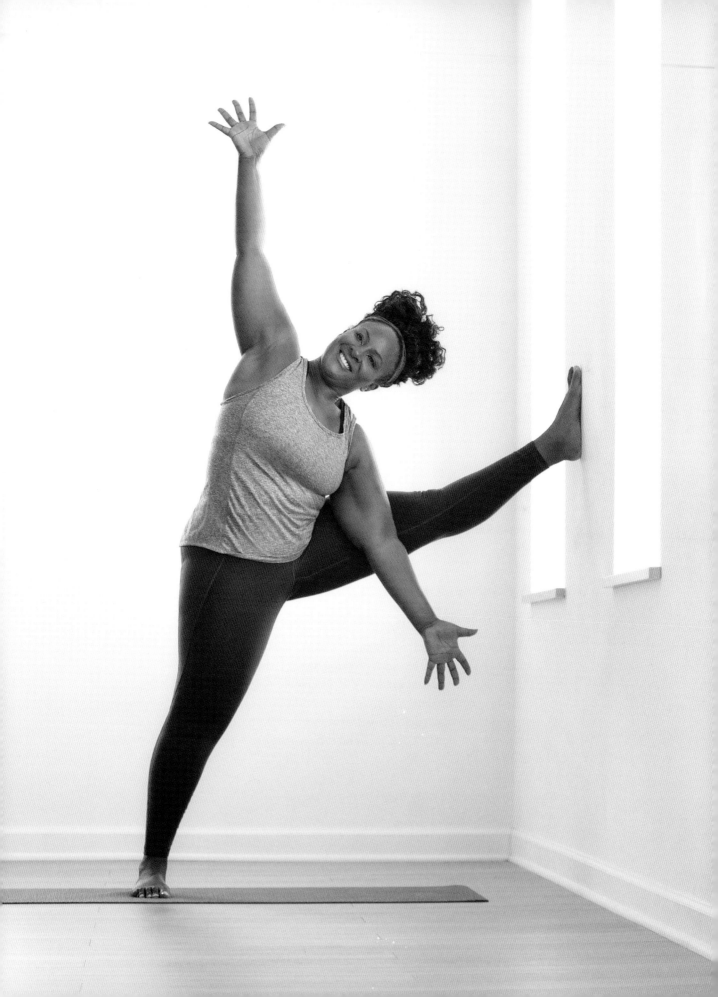

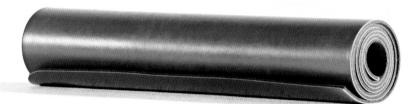

How they vary

You can customize your mat roll as much as you like. In general, if you have a very thick yoga mat you probably won't roll it up all the way, and if your mat is on the thinner side, you might.

Where to find them

Yoga mats are available in lots of places, ranging from your local studio to your local grocery store. And of course, there are tons of options online.

Easy substitutions

For many variations, a rolled-up blanket can take the place of a rolled-up mat— particularly if you want to practice *on* your mat and you don't have an extra one on hand.

BUSTING COMMON MYTHS ABOUT PROPS

Myth #1: Props are just for beginners.

Nope! Props are tools used to facilitate a particular experience in a pose, something that applies to yogis of all levels. A prop might, for example, be used to enhance a specific action (like squeezing a block between your thighs to engage your inner thigh muscles), to accommodate your unique body proportions (no matter how advanced you get, your arms aren't going to get any longer or shorter), to make a pose more restorative (we all need to kick back and relax sometimes), or to make a pose harder (see myth #2).

Myth #2: Props are only used to make poses easier.

Sure, props can be used to make poses easier, and that's great.

    Take a handstand press, for example. This is a very challenging transition where you place your hands on the floor, rise up onto your toes, shift your hips up over your shoulders and push your hands into the ground in order to rise up into a handstand without using any momentum.

Because it can be difficult to get the hips up over the shoulders, lots of people start by standing on yoga blocks, giving the hips a little extra lift from the get-go. After practicing that way for a while to get the hang of the mechanics, they might remove the blocks and try pressing up into a handstand without blocks under their feet. And let's say they do it! And after a while, they're ready for a new challenge. In this case, they might place blocks under their hands, which requires more upper-body strength and makes the press harder!

Or, for another example, try practicing a sun salutation while squeezing a yoga block between your thighs the whole time—and don't let it drop! We're willing to bet that did not make the sun salute easier. In this book we offer all sorts of prop options. Some might make a pose easier for you, others might make the pose harder, and still others might simply make it more interesting.

Myth #3: You're not doing the "full" or "real" form of a pose if you're using a prop.

We want to state this loud and clear: NOPE, NOPE, NOPE, NOPE, NOPE. The "real" version of a pose is whatever version you're doing right now, right here in this reality. The "full" form of a pose is the way in which *you* express the pose most fully, truly making it your own. And the *best* form of a pose is whichever form best serves you.

Myth #4: The best way to make a pose accessible is to use as many props as possible.

As you may have guessed, we love props! And props *are* wonderful tools for making poses more accessible, but more isn't always better. A ton of props can be overwhelming and sometimes unnecessary. The key is to find the props that facilitate the pose experience you're looking for so that you can truly reap its benefits. Sometimes this may mean bringing in several different props, but other times it might be as simple as placing your hands on a wall or rolling up a blanket to place behind your knees. While we know teachers who *love* working with loads of props (and we think that's great if it's your thing), we both tend to think of ourselves as prop minimalists. While we adore props of all kinds, we can get a little flustered working with lots of different props at once and often prefer to see what we can do with one or two props at a time.

Myth #5: The best props cost a lot of money.

We're not gonna lie, yoga props can be expensive, but they don't have to be. When it comes down to it, a blanket is just a blanket, a strap is just a strap, right? Buying the most deluxe version probably isn't going to make your practice any more fulfilling. And the truth is, many yoga props can be replaced with common household items, as we've mentioned, so you don't have to break the bank in order to support your practice.

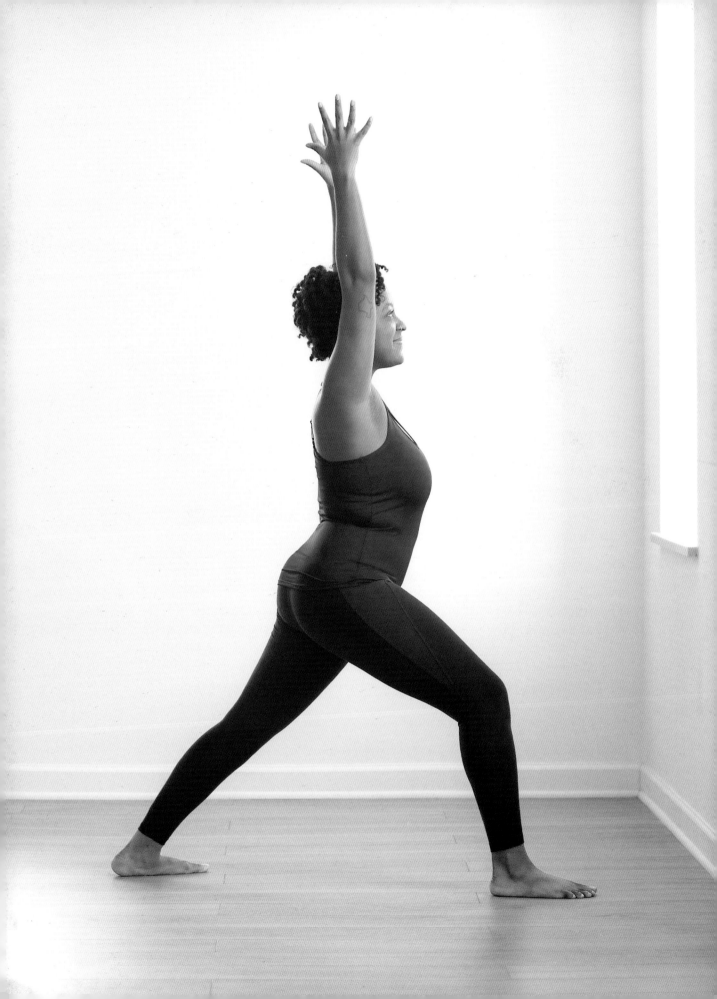

Part Two **THE PRACTICE**

6

Foundational Poses for Vinyasa, Transitions, and Sun Salutes

MOUNTAIN POSE (Tadasana)

Mountain pose is foundational for all standing yoga postures as well as many seated and supine poses and inversions.

Benefits One of the significant benefits of mountain pose is the secure connection between your feet and the earth, giving you a steady foundation to work from. Tadasana can be used to activate and create awareness of the entire body and can improve posture when practiced with intention.

The Practice Stand with your feet comfortably apart, weight equally distributed between both feet and centered over the arches of your feet. Having your feet at "hip distance" or at the distance of your two fists can be a good starting point, but feel free to walk your feet farther apart or closer together if either feels more stable. Your feet can be parallel or slightly turned out, depending on what feels best in your body, but make sure your knees and your toes are pointing in the same direction, aligning your kneecaps with the centers of your ankles.

Keep your arms relaxed at your sides with palms open and turned forward or facing in toward you. Inhale, lengthening your spine up through the crown of your head. Keep that length as you exhale. Keep your gaze forward, your breath steady and even.

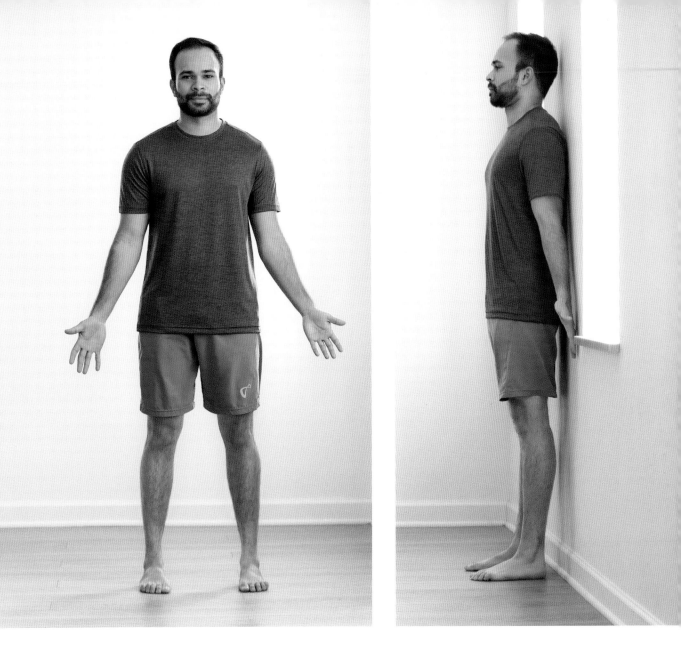

VARIATION 1: AT THE WALL

The wall can be an excellent tool for finding a stable tadasana.

Stand with your back to a wall, your heels a few inches away from it. Align your feet, knees, and ankles just as you would in mountain pose away from the wall.

Bring your bottom, the back of your ribcage, your upper back, the backs of your shoulders, and the back of your head to touch the wall. You may find that you need to walk your feet forward a bit more to do this. You might also find it's more comfortable to bend your knees a little. Note that leaning back against the wall might feel awkward at first because our heads are forward of our shoulders for much of the day as we look at screens, books, the road, and more.

Turn your palms to face forward. Press your feet down into the floor and reach up through the crown of your head.

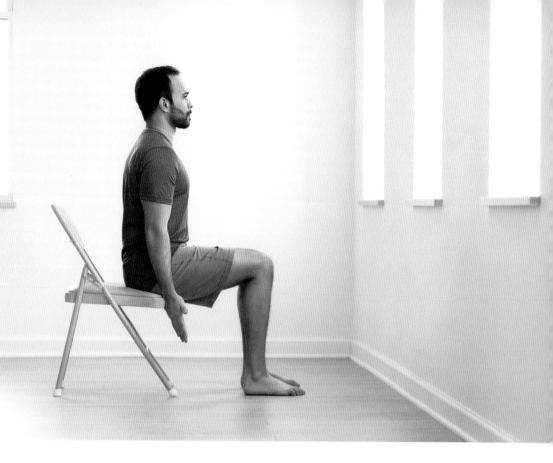

VARIATION 2: SEATED MOUNTAIN POSE

The very definition of *asana* is *seat*. You can be seated and be a mountain. Sit comfortably in a chair with your heels stacked roughly under your knees, feet pressed firmly into the floor, and spine tall. Bring your arms long by your sides with palms turned forward or facing in toward you. Lengthen the sides of your waist and draw your shoulder blades toward each other on your back. Make sure your ears, shoulders, and hips are stacked. Press down through your sitting bones and feet and lengthen up through the top of your head. See if you can sit a little taller as you inhale, and keep that length as you exhale.

TIP If your feet don't touch the floor, place blocks or a bolster under your feet. If you are unable to engage your legs or feet, focus on rooting down through your sitting bones.

VARIATION 3: RECLINED MOUNTAIN POSE (SUPTA TADASANA)

Just like the wall, the floor can provide excellent feedback for your mountain pose. This variation takes gravity out of the equation, making it easier to find a long, neutral spine. This variation also serves as an excellent starting point for any of your supine (reclined) poses (see chapter 13).

Begin lying on your back with the soles of your feet against the wall, feet about hip-distance apart. Turn your palms to face the ceiling (this will help you stay broad through your chest and the fronts of your shoulders).

Notice if your lower ribs are jutting forward, and, if they are, draw them in slightly and lengthen a little more through the back of your ribcage. Press your feet into the wall and reach out through the crown of your head. As in the standing variation of

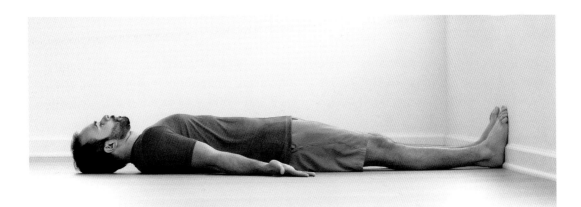

mountain, aim to keep your chin level. If the back of your neck feels compressed, it can be helpful to place a folded blanket or small pillow under your head.

VARIATION 4: UPWARD HAND POSE (URDHVA HASTASANA)

In many vinyasa sequences (including variations of sun salutes), *urdhva hastasana* is the pose we come into before folding forward into *uttanasana* (standing forward bend) and the pose that we return to after rising back up out of uttanasana.

From mountain pose, sweep your arms out to the sides and up alongside your head, turning your palms to face each other. Spin your pinkies toward each other (this can help to soften tension in your neck and shoulders) and keep the back of your head in line with the back of your pelvis.

It may feel better for your neck and shoulders to bring your arms forward a little or a lot. Also experiment with bringing your hands closer together and farther apart and see which position feels best in your body.

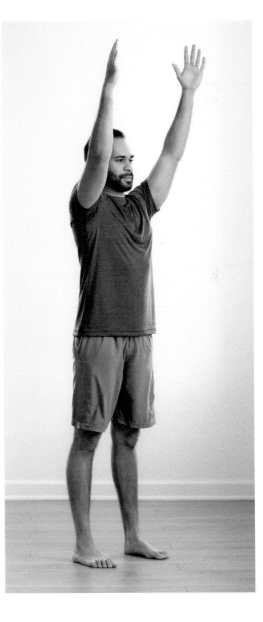

CHAIR POSE (Utkatasana)

Chair pose, or *utkatasana*, is also referred to as "fierce pose" (*utka* means something similar to "fierce" in Sanskrit). Chair pose is often a key component in sun salutes and vinyasa flows since it's a great full-body warm-up and works well as a transitional posture.

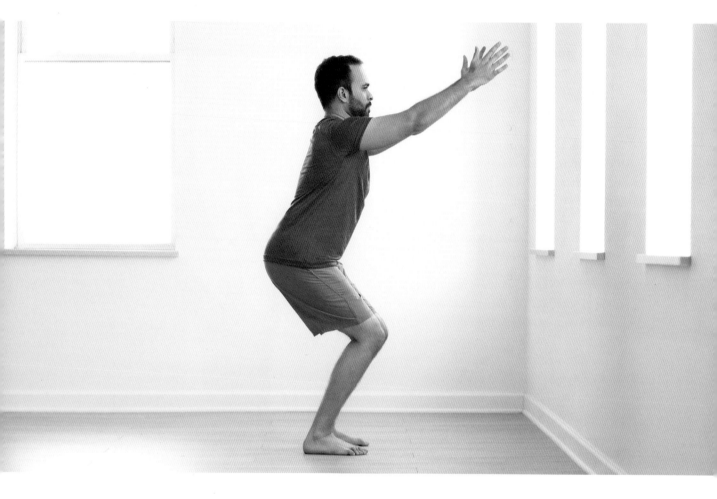

Benefits Chair pose can intensify an asana flow and build endurance.

The Practice Begin standing in mountain pose with weight equally distributed between both feet. If your feet are together with big toes touching, keep a tiny sliver of space between your heels. Keep your knees and toes pointing in the same direction, aligning your kneecaps with the centers of your ankles.

From here, sit your hips back (a little or a lot) as though you were having a seat in a chair. The key to chair pose is not just moving your hips down but moving them back as well.

Glance down and check that your knees aren't going past your toes; if they are, shift a little more weight into your heels, sliding your knees back along with your hips.

Bring your head back to its neutral position, in line with your spine and lift up through your low belly.

You can bring your hands to your heart, reach them forward, reach them up alongside your ears, or into any position that feels good. Stay for three to five breaths, then stand up tall to release.

VARIATION 1: AT THE WALL WITH A BLOCK

The wall provides support and feedback for your chair pose. Squeezing the block helps to engage your inner thighs, pelvic muscles, and deep core muscles and can prevent your knees from dropping inward.

Begin standing in mountain pose facing away from the wall. Start with your heels about a footprint's length away from the wall to begin and adjust as needed as you go. Place a block between your upper inner thighs. Squeeze the block and sit back until your bottom is supported by the wall. Bring your hands to your heart, or reach your arms forward or up. Stay for three to five breaths and then release.

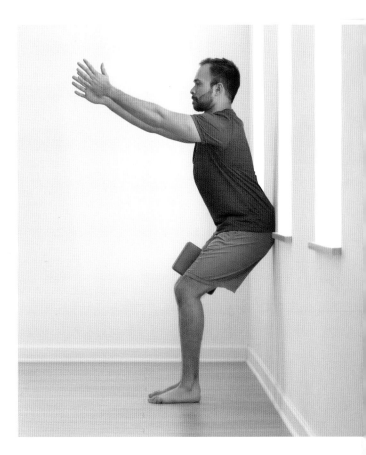

VARIATION 2: WITH HEELS ELEVATED

If you feel a lot of resistance in your ankles when you sit back in chair, or if you just want to experience the posture in a new way, try elevating your heels on a rolled-up yoga mat. This reduces the amount of dorsiflexion required by your ankles, and we think it feels pretty delightful.

Experiment with the thickness of your roll. Unless your mat is very thin, try rolling it up only two-thirds of the way to begin and adjust as needed.

You can also use a rolled-up blanket or towel to elevate your heels.

Stand with your heels up on the roll and the balls of your feet on the floor in front of it, then sit back into chair pose. Notice how this feels in your body. Some people find that this variation feels better for their ankles and that they can sit their hips back a little farther than they can with their feet flat on the floor.

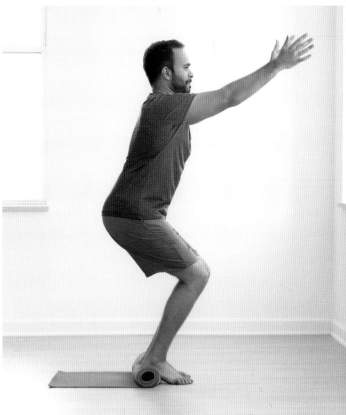

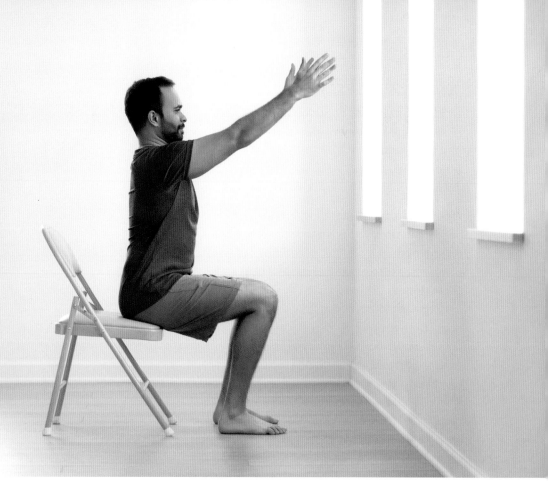

VARIATION 3: IN A CHAIR

Sit on the edge of the chair with your feet flat on the floor and a comfortable distance apart. Press down through your feet so you feel grounded. Root down through your seat, lengthen your spine, and reach your arms forward or up. Remain here or hinge forward and away from the chair, maybe even until your torso is at about a forty-five-degree angle to your seat. Roll your inner upper arms toward each other and stay for three to five breaths. Return to your tall, upright seated position and lower your arms to release.

TIP For an added challenge, try hovering your sitting bones off the chair seat for a breath or two, then lower back down to release.

STANDING FORWARD FOLD (Uttanasana)

Uttanasana, or standing forward fold, is a pose that is also a functional movement—many of us do it every day without thinking about it: we bend over to pick up things from the floor or to put on or tie our shoes. Because of this, an intentional practice of forward folding can go a long way to maintaining back health

Benefits Many yoga practitioners find forward bends to be calming. Uttanasana can also be a great stretch for the hamstrings, glutes, and back.

The Practice Begin standing in mountain pose with your feet a comfortable distance apart. Press down into your feet and resist them apart from each other: pretend they're glued to your mat (so they won't actually move) but you're *trying* to pull them farther apart, and maintain that action. This isometric engagement will activate your outer legs and support you as you fold.

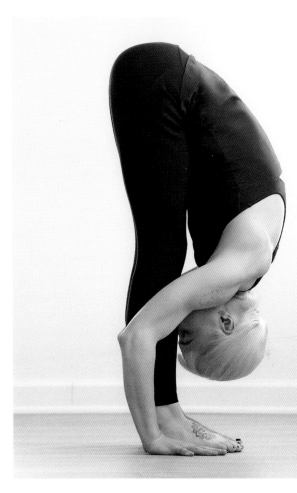

On an inhale, reach up toward the sky, and on an exhale, sweep your arms out to your sides as you hinge forward from your hip creases, bending your knees a little or a lot, and drawing your chest toward your thighs. Keep your spine as long as possible as you fold. Bring your fingertips or hands to the floor or blocks in front of or next to your feet. If there's space between your torso and your thighs (a sign that you're rounding mostly your upper back), bend your knees more until your belly touches your thighs. Relax your head and neck.

Keep your weight over the arches of your feet. Notice if your weight is shifting more into your heels (which is common). What would it feel like to shift more weight into the balls of your feet? Does it change where you feel the stretch in the backs of your legs? Continue pressing down into your feet and resisting them apart from each other. Stay for a few breaths, then sweep your arms out to your sides and rise up to standing with a long spine (bending your knees can help), reaching your arms up overhead when you come up, then bring your arms back alongside you.

TIP If you feel compressed through your midsection or tummy, step your feet out wider to make space for your body. If you feel pulling at your lower or mid back, bend your knees a lot and press your sitting bones back (stick your butt out) to allow your chest to ease forward. Then release your hands to the floor or blocks.

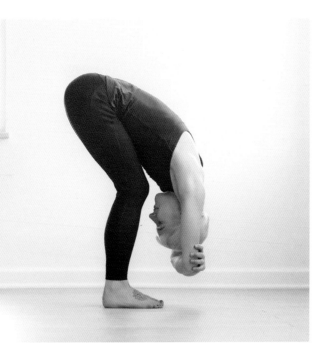

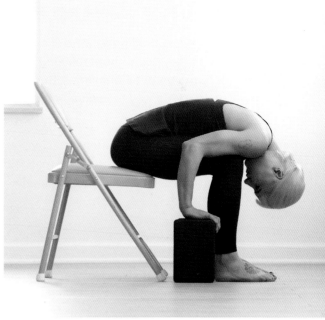

VARIATION 1: DANGLING

This feel-good variation is great if your hamstrings feel tight, and it can be especially nice to do near the beginning or end of your practice, or anytime you want to "hang loose." The key is to keep your torso connected to your thighs, and to maintain an even rounding throughout your spine (i.e., to avoid bringing most of the rounding into your upper back).

From *uttanasana*, bend your knees—a little or a lot, depending on what feels best in your body and allows your torso to connect with your legs if they're not already. Hold on to opposite elbows. Aim to keep your weight evenly distributed through your feet. Lengthen through your neck and allow your head to hang.

Stay for several breaths if you like, then bring your hands to your hips and rise up to standing with a long spine.

VARIATION 2: IN A CHAIR WITH HANDS ON BLOCKS

You will need two blocks and a chair for this variation. Begin in a seated mountain pose (see page 42). Place your blocks on either side of the chair, just in front of the two front chair legs and at their highest setting to begin. Sit tall, near the edge of the seat so that you have room to fold forward. Take your feet out as wide as feels comfortable, perhaps aligning your feet with the chair legs. Inhale your arms up to the sky, and as you exhale sweep them out to the side as you hinge forward from your hip creases, placing your hands on your blocks. If the blocks feel too high, bring them to a lower setting. Aim to find as much length through your spine as you can. Soften your shoulders and release your head and neck toward the floor.

Stay for a few breaths, then rise up to seated with a long spine.

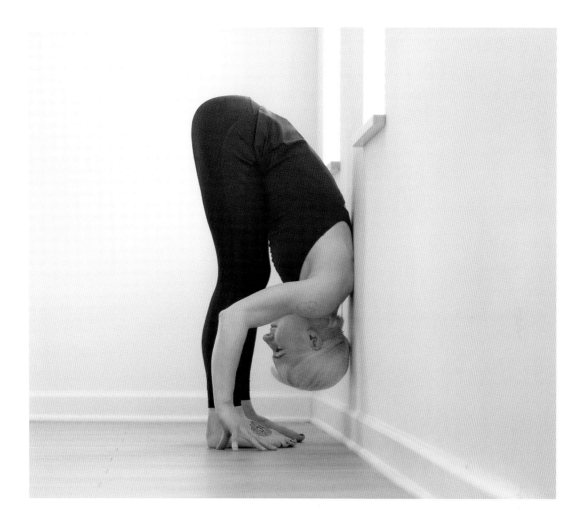

VARIATION 3: STANDING FORWARD BEND AT THE WALL

A wall can provide excellent feedback and support for your standing forward bend and can deepen your experience of the pose.

Stand a few feet away from a wall, facing it, and come into a standing forward bend with your knees bent a little or a lot. From there, walk your hands and feet toward the wall until your upper back and the back of your head touches it. Lightly press your upper back into the wall, and see if you can find a little more length through your spine. This gentle pressure can help to bring some of the rounding out of your upper back and bring a more evenly distributed rounding throughout your whole back. Straighten your legs a little if that feels good. As you explore the pose, adjust your hands and feet as needed (perhaps walking your feet farther apart, closer together, or bringing your hands and feet closer to or farther from the wall).

To come out, step away from the wall so that you have room to come up, bring your hands to your hips, and rise to standing.

CRESCENT LUNGE

In vinyasa yoga in particular, crescent lunge is a staple, often showing up in sun salutations and other flows and serving as a transition between downward-facing dog and standing poses.

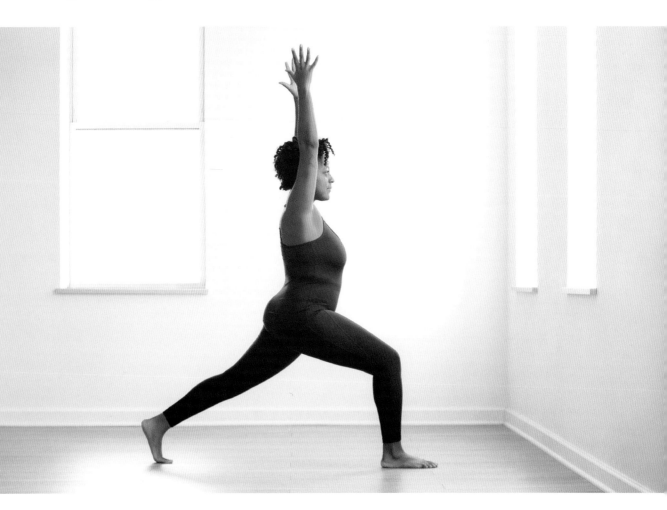

Benefits Crescent lunge can help with balance (precisely because it can be tricky to find your balance). In addition, it stretches the hip flexors of the back leg and engages the glutes and hamstrings of the back leg and the quads of the front leg. Reaching the arms overhead engages your shoulders as well.

The Practice Beginning in standing forward bend at the top of your mat, bend your knees if they're not bent already, then step your left foot back into a lunge.

Keep your entire right foot on the floor and your right knee stacked over your right heel. Keep your left heel lifted and stacked over the ball of your left foot.

Lengthen your spine. Then, bend your back knee a little bit (this will help you to stabilize your pelvis and find more core engagement as you rise up), float your fingertips away from the floor, and lift your torso upright, rising up with both knees bent and then bringing your hands to your hips.

Once you're upright, engage your lower belly: you can think about drawing your two frontal hip bones toward each other, like you're cinching a drawstring, and engaging between your pubic bone and your navel like you're zipping a zipper. Keeping that engagement, and keeping your right knee bent, straighten your left leg, pressing the back of your left thigh up toward the ceiling.

If you like, you can stretch your arms up alongside your ears, or bring them to any position that feels good in your body. Stay for three to five breaths, then lower your hands to the floor and switch sides.

TIP If your balance feels unsteady in crescent lunge or any variations, try walking your forward foot out to the side a little more, widening your stance from side to side, and/or keep your hands on your hips or at heart center. If you want to open the front of the body more, bend your arms into a goal post shape and draw your shoulder blades toward each other to lift your heart forward.

VARIATION 1: WITH A BLOCK AT THE WALL

Crescent lunge can be challenging for the legs and glutes. As a result, there can be a tendency to bend the front knee past the ankle, which can create knee discomfort for some. Using a block and wall for support and resistance is one way to keep your knees feeling great in the pose.

Start facing the wall in mountain pose holding your block in your right hand. Step your left leg back to come into a lunge. Place a block between your right shin and the wall, aligned flush with the wall. Press into the block, and adjust your back leg to a comfortable stance. Align your torso over your hips and lengthen your spine. Reach your arms toward the sky and soften the tops of your shoulders. Hold for three to five breaths, then change sides.

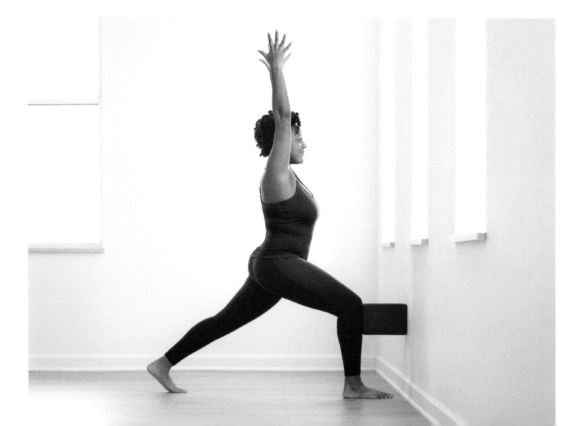

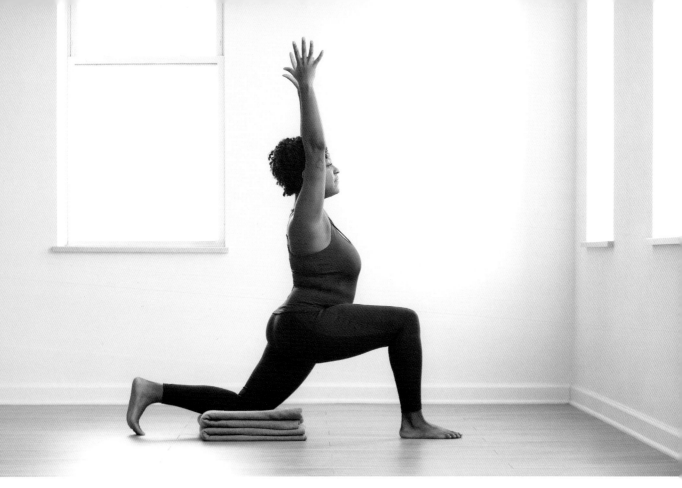

VARIATION 2: BACK KNEE DOWN (*ANJANEYASANA*)[14]

Lowering the back knee to the floor in crescent lunge can often help the pose feel more stable.

Place a blanket or two, folded to your desired thickness, at the back third of your mat, then stand at the top of your mat in uttanasana with your knees bent and your hands or fingertips on the floor or blocks close to your feet.

Step your left leg back into a low lunge, lowering your left knee down onto the blanket and adjusting its positioning as needed. Scoot your left knee back so it's behind your left hip and not directly under it—this will take pressure off of your kneecap.

Your back toes can be tucked under or pointed; see what feels better for your knee.

It's okay for your front knee to go past your ankle if that feels good in your body, but you can also keep your right knee stacked right over your ankle. Make sure that your entire right foot stays on the floor.

Press your fingertips into the floor or blocks, lengthening your spine.

Then, climb your hands up onto your right thigh to bring your torso upright. You can keep your hands on your thigh, bring them to your hips, reach them up overhead, or bring them into any position you like. Stay three to five breaths, then return to uttanasana and change sides.

VARIATION 3: WITH A CHAIR

Start by standing behind the back of a chair. Place both hands on the chair back and step your left foot into a lunge, bending your right knee. You can press your shin against the seat of the chair for extra support. Lengthen your spine and reach your left arm to the sky, keeping your right hand on the chair for balance. Stay three to five breaths, then switch sides.

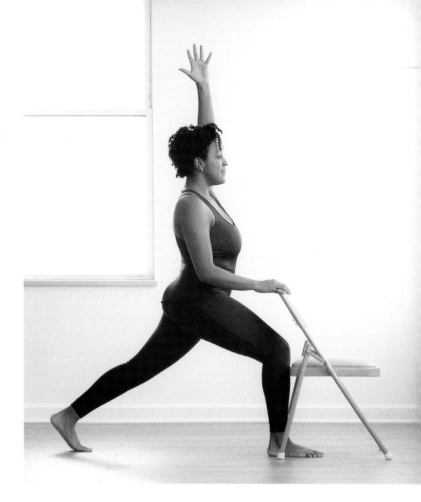

STEPPING INTO A LUNGE FROM DOWNWARD DOG

Though stepping forward into a lunge from downward-facing dog is a common transition in yoga classes, it's not an easy one for many of us. Here are a few different tips for making this tricky transition more accessible.

» Place blocks (on their lowest, flattest setting) underneath your hands in downward dog. This will make your pose a little more spacious and create more room to step forward.

» As you raise a leg and step forward, keep your hips lifted high and, if you're stepping your right foot forward, pop up onto your right fingertips (your left fingertips if you're stepping your left foot forward). This too will create a little more space.

» If you're stepping your right foot forward, pick up your right hand as you step through (your left hand if you're stepping your left foot forward). This also creates space and gives you a little extra momentum to bring your foot to the top of your mat.

» Often, it's easier to step forward into a wider lunge. Instead of stepping your foot between your hands, try stepping your foot outside your hands. (If you're stepping your right foot forward, step outside of your right hand; and if you're stepping your left foot forward, try stepping outside of your left hand.) From here, you could remain in the wide lunge, or walk your front foot between your hands for a narrower one.

» Take as many steps as you need to get your foot between your hands—there's no rule that says you have to do it in one fell swoop! Feel free to bring your hand to your calf/ankle to pick up your foot and move it forward, if that helps.

WARRIOR I (Virabhadrasana I)

Virabhadrasana I is the first of the three warrior poses, but that doesn't mean it's the easiest! Balance and alignment issues can make this ubiquitous asana a challenge for practitioners of all levels.

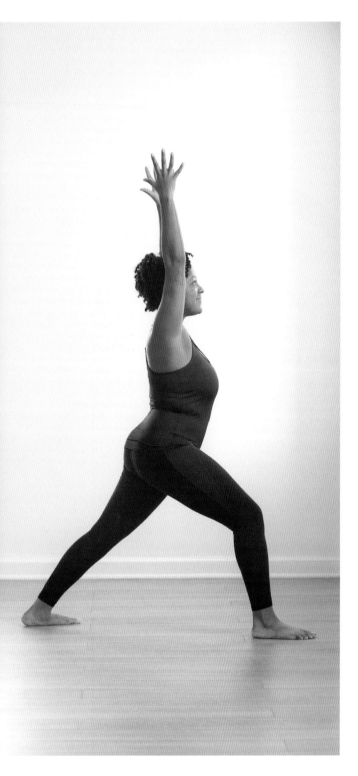

Benefits Truly a "full body" pose, warrior I stretches the hip flexors of the back leg and engages the hamstrings and glutes of the back leg and the quads of the front leg. It also engages the muscles of the shoulders when you lift your arms up.

The Practice While there are many ways to come into warrior I pose, it's often first taught from mountain pose, so we'll look at that version to start.

Begin in mountain pose with your feet hip-width apart or slighter wider. Step your left leg back, about a leg's length, and bring your whole left foot to the floor, with your left toes slightly turned out so that they're pointing toward the upper left corner of your mat.

If you feel unstable, walk your right foot a little to the right, widening your stance from side to side.

Keeping your left foot grounded, bend your right knee so that it's stacked over your right ankle, aiming your kneecap in the same direction as the center of your ankle.

Press down evenly through both of your feet. If your back heel is lifting away from the floor, you can place a rolled blanket or rolled mat underneath it, or you can step your left foot forward a little, shortening your stance from front to back, or you can let your back toes turn out more. See what feels best in your body.

Your front thigh does not need to be at a "perfect" ninety-degree angle, but if you'd like to increase the strength work required of your front leg, you can walk your left foot back a little more, lengthening your stance from front to back so that you can bend your front knee more deeply.

Don't worry about making your hips square to the front of the mat—often attempting to do so will cause you to twist your back knee, which might not feel so great. It's okay for your hips to open up to the left a bit—for most of us that will be the case!

Once you've found your ideal warrior I position, reach your arms up alongside your ears (or bring them more forward if that feels better for you). Spin your pinkies in toward each other to release tension in your neck and shoulders.

Stay three to five breaths, then change sides.

VARIATION: IN A CHAIR

In this chair-enhanced variation of warrior I, we have also added a mat to support the back heel. You'll want an armless chair for this one.

Start by straddling your right leg over the chair, positioning your right thigh, so it is supported by the seat of the chair. Make sure your thigh feels fully supported and your knee is bent with the edge of the seat supporting the back of the knee. Extend your left leg behind you. Support your left thigh with the seat of the chair, and turn your left toes out slightly to the left. Make sure the position of your back leg feels good for your knee. It can be challenging to get your back foot flat on the floor in this variation (as your stance is longer than a non-chair-enhanced warrior I), so you may wish to use a rolled mat (as shown), a rolled or folded blanket, or a yoga block to support your left heel.

Once you feel stable, press down into the seat with your legs, press out through your feet, and reach your arms up, squaring your shoulders forward. Stay for three to five breaths, then change sides.

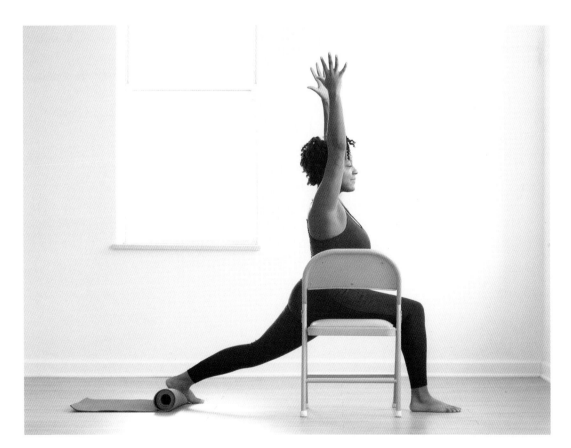

COBRA POSE (Bhujangasana)

Cobra is often one of the first backbends people learn in yoga. It gets its name from its resemblance to the hood of a cobra as it's raising its head to strike. Cobra plays an important role in sun salutes, as it's often done in place of, or in preparation for, upward-facing dog pose (see page 58).

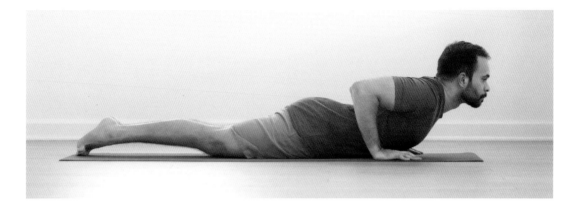

Benefits Cobra stretches the shoulders, chest, and abdominals. It's an excellent preparation for deeper backbends and a great pose to include in a warm-up and after abdominal-strengthening work.

The Practice Begin lying on your belly with your legs long and the tops of your feet pressing into the floor. You can also curl your toes under if it feels better. Bend your elbows and place your hands beside your chest on either side of your body. Hug your elbows into the sides of your body (but not so much that your shoulders round forward).

Press down through the tops of your feet and your pubic bone. Resist the heels of your hands toward the back of your mat and, on an inhale, lift your chest and head away from the floor. Keep your lower ribs on the floor.

Squeeze your shoulders blades together, broaden your chest, and lengthen up through your crown. Gaze forward like you're looking over the edge of a precipice. Aim to use your back muscles (not your hands) to hold you up. You can even lift your hands away from the floor to see if you can maintain your lift without them.

Stay here, or, for a deeper backbend, place your hands back down, resist the heels of your hands toward the back of your mat again, and see if you can lift a little higher, perhaps lifting your low ribs away from the floor but keeping your pelvis and thighs on the floor.

Stay three to five breaths, then, on an exhale, lower your chest and head back to the mat.

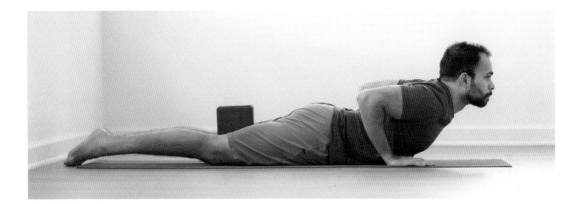

VARIATION 1: WITH A BLOCK

To keep your low back from taking on too much of the work and to help you engage your deep core muscles, place a block between your thighs. Squeeze the block as you lift into cobra.

VARIATION 2: AT THE WALL

This is a great variation to work with if lying on your belly is contraindicated or uncomfortable for you.

Begin by standing facing a wall and bring your toes to touch the baseboard. Your pelvis, chest, and hands will be touching the wall. Bring your hands to the wall at chest height. Root down into your feet, keep your pelvis on the wall, and on an inhale, curl your shoulders back and lift your chest away from the wall to come into a cobra shape. Engage your upper back by squeezing your shoulder blades together and broadening your chest more. Gaze up to where the wall meets the ceiling. Stay three to five breaths, then return to your starting position.

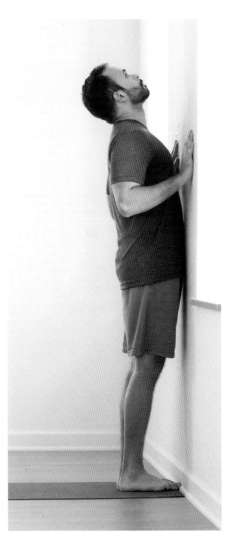

UPWARD-FACING DOG POSE (Urdhva Mukha Svanasana)

Though upward-facing dog is well known in sun salutations, this backbend is worth exploring as a stand-alone pose too. It differs from cobra (see previous pose) in that your arms are straight and your thighs are lifted away from the floor.

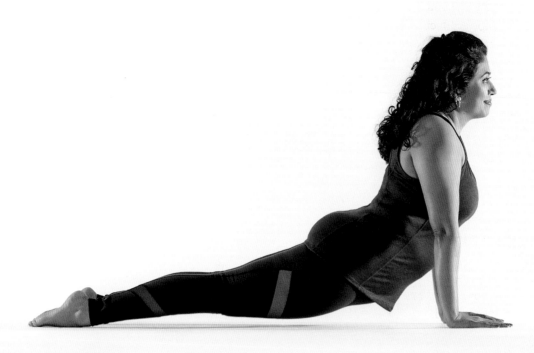

Benefits Upward-facing dog engages the back of the body and opens the front of the body, offering up a nice stretch for the abdomen, chest, and shoulders. It can feel particularly good after abdominal work. It also provides a nice stretch for the tops of your feet.

The Practice Though upward-facing dog is often entered via *chaturanga* (see page 68), let's first explore it from the ground up.

Up-Dog from the Ground Up

Begin lying on your belly. Bend your elbows and walk your hands back so that your wrists are under your elbows. Your forehead can rest on the floor or hover above it. Reach back through your legs and press all of your toenails—even your pinky toenails— into the floor. Lift the fronts of your shoulders away from the floor. On an inhale, lift your chest to come into cobra. Then, lift your thighs away from the floor. Keep your chest broad as you start to straighten your arms. Keep your gaze straight ahead or allow your head to move back slightly, following the movement of the backbend.

Stay for three breaths, then either lower back down to your belly or tuck your toes under and press back to downward dog.

TIP Keeping a microbend in your elbows may help you access more chest expansion and take stress off of your lower back.

If your shoulders aren't in line with your wrists when you come up, lower back onto your belly and start over with your hands a little more forward or farther back as needed.

Up-Dog from Plank

Did you know that you can skip chaturanga in sun salutations and move directly from plank into upward-facing dog? Here's how: From plank (see page 65), flip onto the tops of your feet one at a time (start with the right). Then, without touching your thighs or pelvis to the floor, lower your pelvis *toward* the floor and broaden and lift your chest to come into upward dog. Exit the pose by tucking your toes (one at a time, or by rolling over the tops of your feet) to come into downward-facing dog. The next time you come into up-dog, start by flipping onto the top of your left foot first. And if you tucked your toes under one at a time to come into downward dog, alternate your lead foot there as well.

Up-Dog from Chaturanga

If you're coming into upward-facing dog from chaturanga (see page 68), pause in chaturanga with your shoulders lifted higher than your elbows and your chest broad—at a point where you could press back up into plank if you needed to. From there, either roll over the tops of your feet to come into upward dog or untuck your toes one at a time. Keep your thighs lifting away from the floor, your pelvis moving toward the floor, and your chest broad. Stay for a few breaths or move right back to downward dog.

TIP Depending on your proportions, rolling over the tops of your feet to come into upward dog from chaturanga might cause you to end up with your shoulders past your wrists in upward dog, which isn't super comfortable. If that's the case, you can simply slide your feet back so that your shoulders are right over your wrists, or you can untuck your toes one at a time to move into up-dog instead of rolling over both feet at once. See what feels best in your body.

VARIATION 1: AT THE WALL

Begin standing about arm distance away from the wall with feet roughly hip-width apart and parallel. Place your hands on the wall, just below shoulder height, then walk your feet back about a step or so. Press your hands into the wall and, keeping your arms long and strong, curl your shoulders back, broaden your chest, and lift your gaze toward the ceiling. Stay for three to five breaths, then continue to press into the wall as you return to starting position.

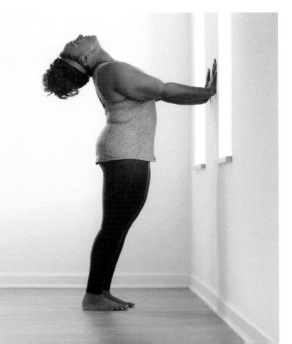

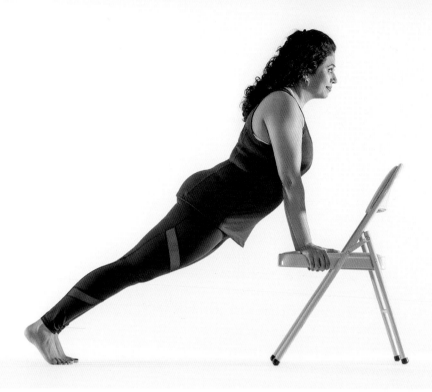

VARIATION 2: ON A CHAIR

Up-dog can be challenging for the arms, tops of the feet, and the lower back. One way to build strength and to create a more accessible variation of this pose is to use a chair.

Begin standing about a foot in front of the chair, facing the seat. Fold forward and grasp the outer edges of the seat. Walk your feet back until you are in a plank position, making a long diagonal line from heels to crown. Firm your core, and keeping your arms straight, draw your heart forward through your arms, broadening your chest as you look over the top of the back of the chair. You can gaze upward slightly if that feels comfortable for your neck. Stay three to five breaths. To release, press back to your chair-supported plank (or a chair-supported downward dog, see page 63), then walk your feet in toward the chair.

VARIATION 3: ON A BOLSTER

This is a great variation to try if your arms are on the shorter side or you find it challenging to lift your thighs away from the floor in upward dog.

Begin lying face down on the bolster. Align your lower ribs with the top edge of the bolster. Separate your feet a close yet comfortable distance with the tops of your feet pressing into the floor. (You can also tuck your toes under if you like.) Place your hands on either side of the bolster and walk them back so that your wrists are under your elbows. From here, begin to curl your chest forward as you straighten your arms and lift your torso from the bolster, keeping your pelvis and thighs supported. Gaze forward or slightly up if that feels good for your neck. Stay three to five breaths, then release back down onto the bolster.

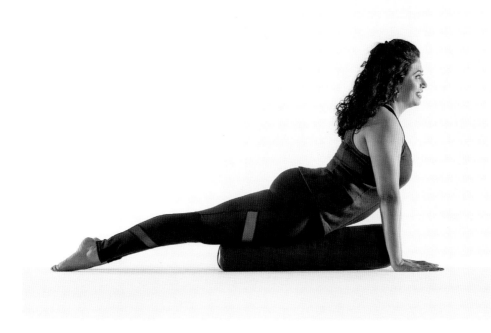

VARIATION 4: ON BLOCKS

As with the bolster-supported variation, practicing with your hands on blocks can make up-dog feel a lot more spacious, and may help you to access the backbend more readily.

To try it, come into plank with your hands on blocks (on their flattest setting) and come into upward-facing dog via chaturanga or plank as you typically would. See how much more room you have to work with! When you're done, press back into a block-supported downward dog.

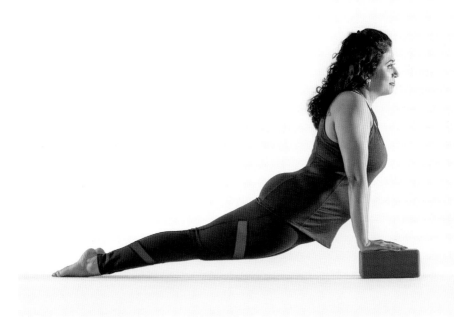

DOWNWARD-FACING DOG POSE (Adho Mukha Svanasana)

Downward dog is one of the most recognizable yoga poses. It's an integral part of sun salutations and is often done many times during a yoga class as a transition between different poses.

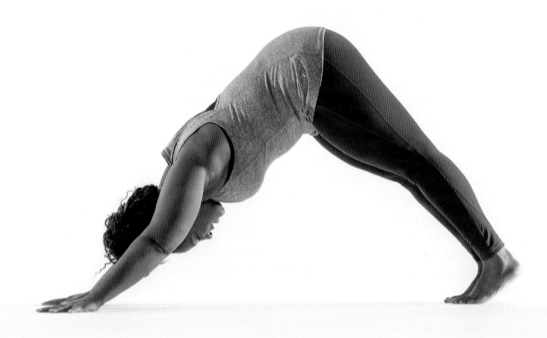

Benefits Downward dog is a weight-bearing, strength-building pose that engages the shoulders and arms while stretching the glutes, hamstrings, calves, and back. Because your head is below your heart, downward dog is technically an inversion, and it's a key preparation for more challenging inversions like handstand.

The Practice Begin on hands and knees with your toes tucked under. Walk each of your hands one handprint in front of your shoulders. Make sure your hands are shoulder-width apart (or slightly wider) and the creases of your wrists are parallel with the top edge of your mat. Spread your fingers a comfortable distance. Inhale here, and, on an exhale, lift your knees and press your hips up and back to make the shape of a big inverted V. Press the floor away with your hands, and press your thighs back to begin to straighten your legs. They don't need to straighten all the way; if your back begins to round, that's a sign to bend your knees more.

Relax your head and neck, taking your gaze toward the center of your mat or back toward your toes, whichever feels best for your neck.

Stay for several breaths, then release by bringing your knees back to the floor.

VARIATION 1: WITH HANDS ON BLOCKS

In this variation, blocks lengthen your arms and create more space to expand your chest.

Begin on hands and knees with your blocks under your hands at either their flattest or middle setting (experiment to see what feels best). If you like, you can grip the edges of the blocks with your fingers and thumbs. Once your hands are in place, tuck your toes, lift your knees, and press your hips back into downward-facing dog. Walk your feet back as needed to find a down-dog length that works for you.

VARIATION 2: ON A CHAIR SEAT

Start facing the seat of the chair. Come to a forward fold placing your hands on the seat of the chair. Your fingers can wrap around the edges of the seat for stability if you like. Walk your feet back behind you, lengthening your arms and your spine to come into a down-dog position. Keep your head in line with your spine and your neck long. Root down through your heels and rotate your upper arms in toward your ears. You may wish to bend your knees in order to keep your spine long. Stay for several breaths, then walk your feet forward to come out of the pose.

VARIATION 3: ON A CHAIR BACK

Sometimes you need a little more height for your chair dog. Using the chair back instead of the chair seat will give you just that! Face the back of the chair and hold on to it firmly with both hands. As in the previous variation, walk your feet back behind you, lengthening your arms and your spine to find your downward dog. Align the back of your head with the back of your pelvis to keep your head in line with your spine. Bend your knees if that helps you find more length through your spine. Walk your feet forward to come out of the pose when you're done.

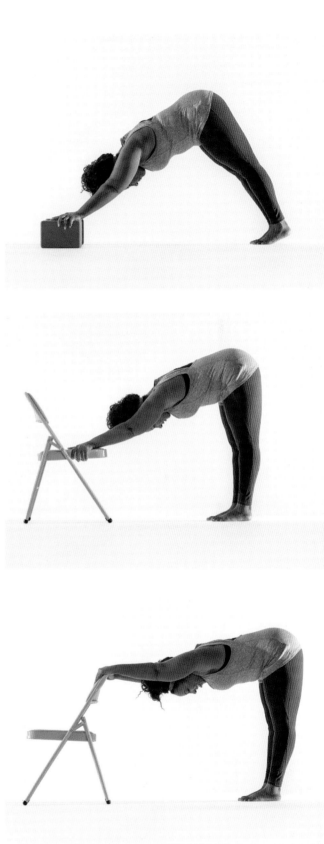

VARIATION 4: AT THE WALL

Place your hands on the wall with your arms straight. Arrange your hands so that they're shoulder-width apart with your wrist creases making a straight line and your fingers spread a comfortable distance apart. If you'd like to come into more of an L shape at the wall, your wrist creases will be a little below shoulder height. To make more of a V shape, with your spine slanted upward at a diagonal, have your hands at or above shoulder height (both versions have their advantages. Experiment and see what best suits your needs).

Walk your feet back, bringing your heels beneath your hips. Keep your ears roughly in line with your biceps (avoid dropping your head or lifting your chin; keep your neck long and reach out through your crown). Roll your inner upper arms upward. Your aim is to find as much length through your spine as possible, so you may find it helpful to bend your knees. Press your hands into the wall and reach back through your hips. Stay for several breaths, then walk your feet toward the wall and your hands up the wall to come out, releasing your arms alongside you when you're done.

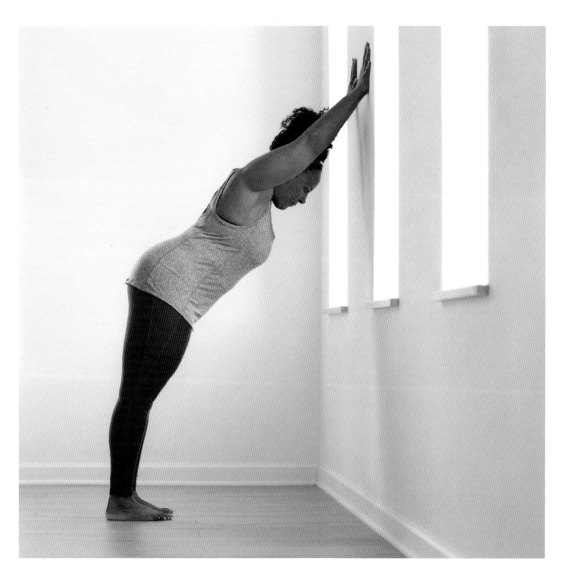

PLANK POSE

(Kumbhakasana, Phalakasana, or Adho Mukha Dandasana)

Plank is simple but not easy. Plank is often used as a transitional pose in sun salutations and other vinyasa flows.

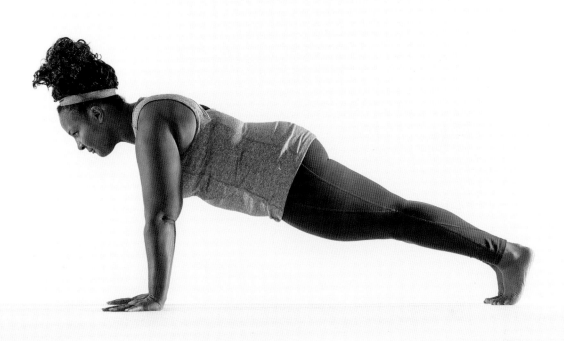

Benefits Plank builds strength in the arms, shoulders, wrists, and hands. It also strengthens the legs, the abdominals, and the back muscles. It's an essential preparation for arm-balancing poses, and holding it is a great way to build endurance!

The Practice Begin on hands and knees, with your fingers spread a comfortable distance apart. For more stability, take your hands a little wider than your shoulders with the pinky fingers aligning with the outer shoulders. Keep your neck long, gazing between your hands. Tuck your toes and step your feet back, making a straight line with your body from head to heels.

Keep your hips and thighs lifted as you reach back through your inner heels. Keep your head in line with your spine. Stay three to five breaths, then lower your knees to the floor to release.

VARIATION 1: FOREARM PLANK

If you want to bear less weight through your hands and wrists (or if you just want to mix things up!) try plank on your forearms. Keep your shoulders stacked over your elbows. You can keep your forearms parallel—which can help you to stay broad through your chest and is an excellent prep for forearm balance (see page 157)—or with your hands clasped or in a prayer position. You could also hold a block between your hands, which can prevent your elbows from splaying.

TIP One way to keep your mind occupied—and to mobilize your shoulders while you're at it—is to shift forward and back. For example: inhale and shift your weight forward, coming more onto your toes and bringing your shoulders past your elbows; exhale and shift back, reaching through your heels and bringing your shoulders behind your elbows. This is especially helpful when you're holding plank for a set time (say, thirty seconds). Give it a try, and watch those seconds fly by!

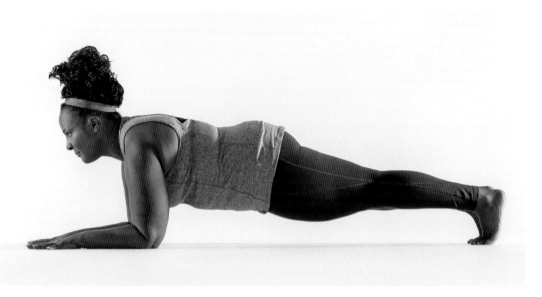

VARIATION 2: KNEES-DOWN PLANK

Try this variation if you tend to drop your hips and arch your lower back in plank or if you're going to be holding plank for a long time. It's also a nice stop between plank and chaturanga (see page 68), allowing you to maintain more control and core engagement as you lower. To come into it, you can begin in a knees-up plank, then lower your knees toward the floor without moving them forward or back. Your toes can remain tucked, or you can point them.

You can also come into kneeling plank from all fours: without changing anything else, slide your knees back so that instead of being directly under your hips, they're behind them.

VARIATION 3: CHAIR PLANK

Begin by standing in front of the seat of a chair. Place both hands on the seat of the chair and wrap your fingers around the sides of the seat for support. Walk your feet back so that your body creates a straight line. Come up onto your toes and press back through your heels. Take your gaze over the back of the chair.

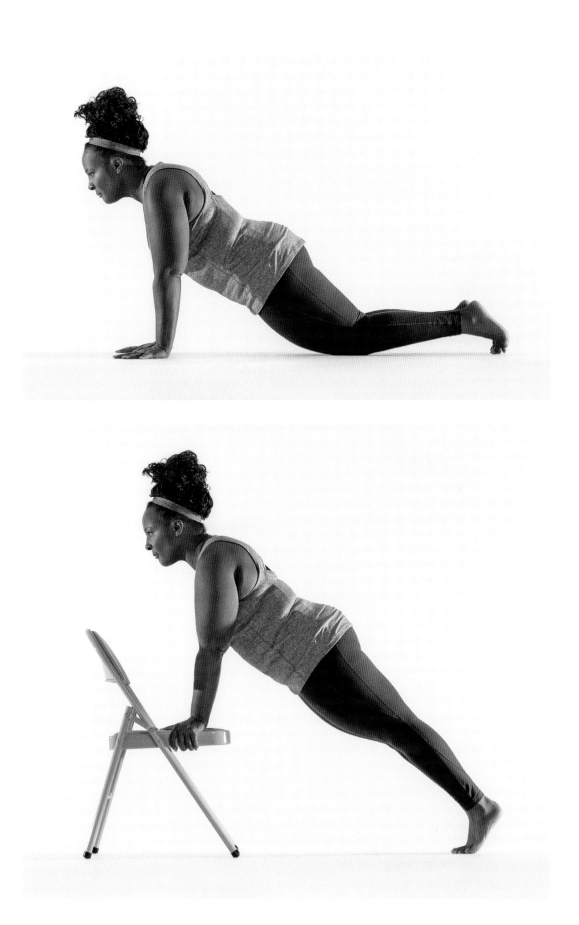

FOUR-LIMBED STAFF POSE (Chaturanga Dandasana)

Chaturanga is *very* familiar to most vinyasa yoga practitioners. If you practice a lot of sun salutes and flows, odds are you're going to be doing a lot of chaturanga (though today, recognizing the importance of varying our movement, many teachers are offering fewer chaturangas and more alternatives). Chaturanga, also known as four-limbed staff pose, doesn't always have to look a certain way. The "right" way to practice chaturanga is the way that feels best in your body and supports your needs and goals.

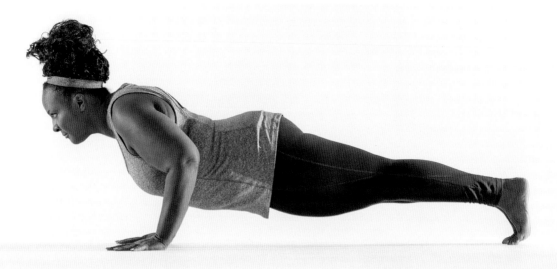

Benefits When practiced regularly, chaturanga can cultivate core and shoulder stability and strength. It's also a fabulous preparation for arm balances, as many arm-balancing asanas require a chaturanga-like position in the upper body.

The Practice From plank (see page 65), shift forward onto the balls of your feet so your shoulders move forward of your wrists. This will help you maintain even weight distribution through your shoulders, elbows, and wrists as you lower. Keeping your chest and the fronts of your shoulders broad, bend your elbows. Keep your elbows pointing back (instead of out to the sides like a push-up), but don't squeeze them into your ribs so tightly that it causes your shoulders to round. Bend your elbows a little or a lot, and see how it feels to keep your shoulders *higher* than your elbows in chaturanga (this means you won't come to a ninety-degree angle). Ultimately, whether you come to a ninety-degree angle or lower or keep your shoulders above your elbows depends on many factors, including whether or not you are working with or recovering from an injury, the number of chaturangas you're doing, your practice goals and intentions, and your unique body proportions. If you are practicing a lot of chaturangas, keeping your shoulders higher than your elbows may make for a more sustainable chaturanga.

From chaturanga, you could hold for a few breaths if you're feeling adventurous, or transition into an upward-facing dog, or press up into plank pose again, or lower all the way down to your belly.

VARIATION 1: KNEES-DOWN CHATURANGA

Lowering your knees in chaturanga can make it easier to refine the actions of the pose, allowing you to explore it with enhanced stability and control.

When coming into this one, think of what will make it easiest for you to shift your shoulders past your wrists. You could start in a knees-up plank pose, shift forward, and then lower your knees; or you could lower your knees first and then shift forward. See what feels best in your body. If you're transitioning onto your belly for cobra or into up-dog, you may want to point your toes, which can allow for a smoother transition.

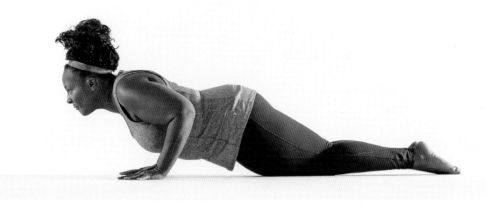

VARIATION 2: WITH HANDS ON BLOCKS

Chaturanga with hands on blocks is a great variation to try if you have sore wrists because it changes the weight distribution, recruiting more engagement of the chest muscles and taking strain out of the wrists.

Start on hands and knees with fingers wrapped around blocks that are on their lowest or medium setting. Align the blocks underneath your shoulders with the top edges aligning with the tops of your shoulders. Press down into the blocks and extend one leg at a time to come into a plank. Then, on an exhale, bend your elbows and bring your upper arms alongside your body for chaturanga.

From here, on an inhale, you can press right back up to plank or transition into a block-supported upward-facing dog and then exhale into a block-supported downward-facing dog.

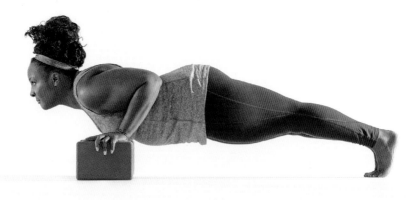

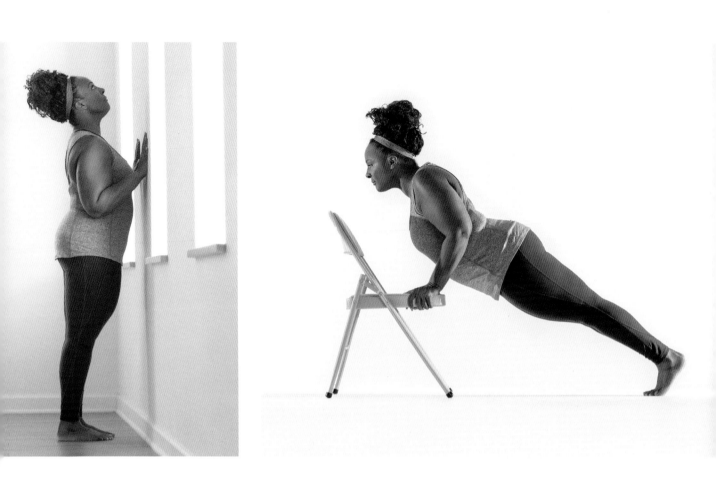

VARIATION 3: AT THE WALL

This is one of the most accessible versions of this pose because it distributes the weight more evenly through the feet and hands.

Stand about a foot away from the wall. Place your hands on the wall at shoulder height, shoulder-distance apart. Set up so that your outer shoulders align with your pinky fingers and your fingertips align with the tops of your shoulders. Inhale here, and, on an exhale, bend your elbows and lower your torso toward the wall. Staying broad through your chest, hug your elbows in toward your ribs so that your arms are parallel to your torso. Lift your gaze slightly if that feels good for your neck.

On an inhale, straighten your arms and then release them back down to your sides.

VARIATION 4: WITH A CHAIR

This is a great variation for building strength and/or if you have difficulty moving up from and down to the floor. Using a chair can also be more wrist-friendly because it changes the angle in which you distribute weight through your wrists.

Begin standing in front of the seat of a chair. Hold on to the seat, wrapping your fingers around the edges. Walk your feet back so that your body creates a straight line, coming into a chair-supported plank. On an exhale, bend your elbows so they are alongside your torso and your chest lowers toward the chair. Stay broad through your chest and reach back through your heels. Take your gaze over the back of the chair. Straighten your arms on an inhale, and walk your feet back in toward the chair to come out.

COMMON SUN SALUTATIONS

Though there are many sun salute variations, these are two that incorporate many of the poses in this chapter and that you are likely to come across in some form or another in a typical vinyasa-style yoga class:

SUN SALUTATION A
(Surya Namaskar A)

» Begin in mountain pose

» Inhale, upward salute

» Exhale, standing forward bend

» Inhale, half-standing forward bend (sometimes cued as "flat back")

» Exhale, standing forward bend

» Inhale, plank

» Exhale, chaturanga (*Note:* you can also jump right back to chaturanga from half-standing forward bend)

» Inhale, upward-facing dog (or cobra)

» Exhale, downward-facing dog (hold for a few breaths)

» Inhale, rise up onto the balls of your feet; exhale, bend your knees, and gaze forward, and step or jump to standing forward bend

» Inhale, half-standing forward bend

» Exhale, standing forward bend

» Inhale, rise to stand, sweeping your arms out to the sides and up

» Exhale, return to mountain pose with hands at heart

SUN SALUTATION B
(Surya Namaskar B)

» Begin in mountain pose

» Inhale, chair pose

» Exhale, standing forward bend

» Inhale, half-standing forward bend

» Exhale, standing forward bend

» Inhale, plank

» Exhale, chaturanga (or jump right back to chaturanga from half-standing forward bend)

» Inhale, upward-facing dog (or cobra)

» Exhale, downward-facing dog

» Inhale, warrior I with right foot forward (or take a few breaths to get there if you'd rather)

» Exhale, chaturanga

» Inhale, upward-facing dog

» Exhale, downward-facing dog

» Inhale, warrior I with left foot forward

» Exhale, chaturanga

» Inhale, upward-facing dog

» Exhale, downward-facing dog (hold for a few breaths)

» Inhale, rise up onto the balls of your feet; exhale, bend your knees, and gaze forward, and step or jump to standing forward bend

» Inhale, half-standing forward bend

» Exhale, standing forward bend

» Inhale, chair pose

» Exhale, return to mountain pose with hands at heart

7

Standing Poses

WARRIOR II (Virabhadrasana II)

We love a warrior pose because it reminds us to stand in our power so we can shine our light into the world.

Benefits Warrior II is a great pose for building endurance, and it strengthens the muscles of the thighs and buttocks. It also requires you to engage your shoulders (when your arms are outstretched), abdominals, ankles, and the arches of your feet.

The Practice Stand facing the long side of your mat with your feet wide apart. Stretch your arms out to a T position and if possible, align your wrists over your ankles. This is just a reference point for the width of your feet; bring your hands back to your hips once you've found your wide stance.

Turn your right foot out, so your toes point to the top of your mat. Make the outer edge of your left foot parallel with the back edge of your mat, or turn your back toes in slightly (the back foot tends to turn out in warrior II, so erring on the side of turning it in a little can be helpful).

"Traditionally" this pose is taught with the heel of the front foot lined up with the arch of the back foot, but for many of us, that stance is too narrow, making it difficult to balance. As such, many people find it helpful to align the front heel with the back heel instead. Experiment to find a position that works for you.

Bring your arms back to a T position, raising them out to your sides at shoulder height so they're parallel to the floor. Make sure your torso is aligned over your hips (not leaning forward or back).

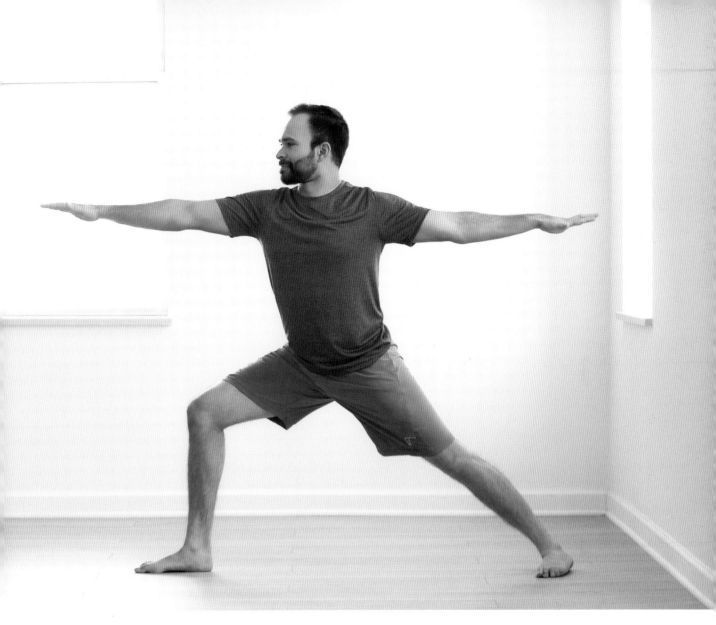

Bend your right knee to align over your right ankle. If your right knee is forward of your ankle and that doesn't feel good, back off a little (bend your front knee less) or widen your stance. Keep in mind that your front thigh doesn't need to be at a "perfect" ninety-degree angle. If the pose feels too intense for your front thigh, try shortening your stance.

Track your right knee toward the center of your right foot. There's a tendency for the knee to collapse inward, toward the big-toe side of the foot, particularly if your hips are tight. To counter this, keep the ball of your right big toe grounded and aim your right knee toward the pinky-toe side of your right foot.

Turn your head to the right and gaze out across the tip of your right middle finger. Press your feet down and apart from each other, as though you were trying to stretch your mat apart, to stabilize your leg. Stay three to five breaths, then change sides.

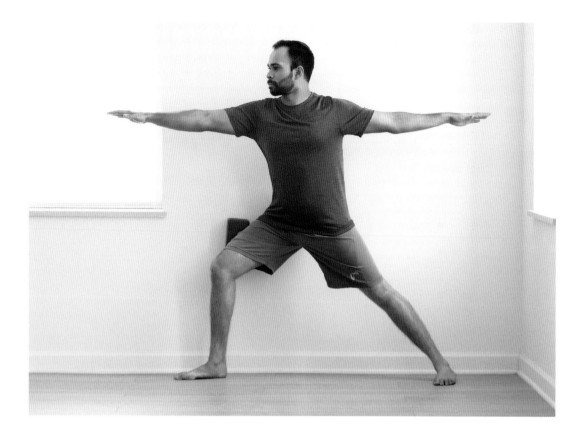

VARIATION 1: AT THE WALL WITH A BLOCK

This is a great variation if your front knee tends to roll in, toward the big-toe side of your foot in warrior II. Working with a block against a wall can help you to engage your front hip's external rotators and keep your front knee tracking in line with the center of your front foot.

Set up for warrior II on the right with your back facing a wall, close enough to the wall that your left heel is touching it. Place your block—on its narrowest or medium setting—between your right knee or thigh and the wall. Whether your block is the narrow way or the medium way will depend on how close your right foot is to the wall. Your goal is to have your right knee pointing toward the center of your right foot, so adjust your block placement and/or stance if needed.

Root down into the ball of your right big toe and press into the block, pushing it into the wall. See if you can feel your right hip muscles engage as you do this. Stay for three to five breaths, then switch sides.

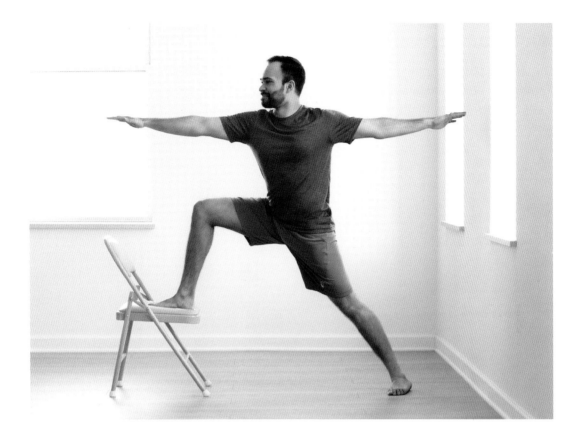

VARIATION 2: FRONT FOOT ON A CHAIR

We love this variation, which we learned from our very creative friend, fellow yoga teacher Allison Jeraci. Why? Because it brings more load (work) into the back leg and lets us experience the pose in a totally different way.

Place the chair at the top of your mat with the seat facing you.

Hold on to the chair to aid in your balance as you step your right foot up onto the seat (knee stacked over ankle) and walk your left foot back into warrior II position. Stretch your arms out to a T, opening up to face the long edge of your mat. Keep your back foot grounded.

TIP Though in the picture Jai is playing fast and loose without a mat in the photo, we recommend having all four chair legs on a mat. The added grip will keep it from sliding, which will keep *you* from doing an accidental split!

If the chair feels unstable, place it against a wall (with the back of the chair against the wall). If your foot is slipping off of the chair, place a folded yoga mat on the seat for added grip.

WARRIOR III (Virabhadrasana III)

The warrior poses inspire us to remember our capacity for strength, stamina, and focus. And warrior III, in particular, can really challenge our balance. It can also make us feel like we're flying, perhaps that's why it's also referred to as "airplane pose" when practiced with arms alongside the body instead of reaching forward or at heart center.

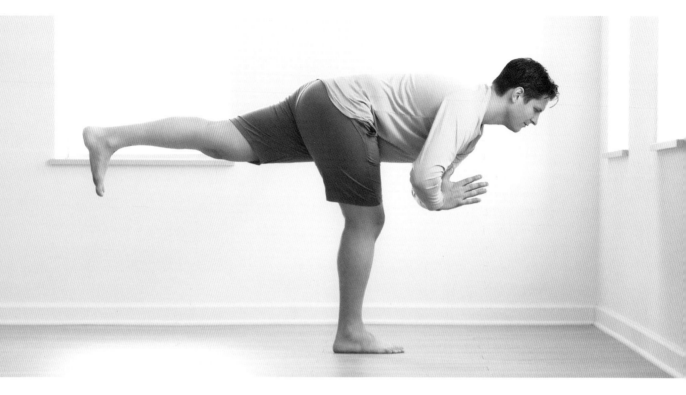

Benefits Warrior III activates the legs and core muscles and can improve balance and proprioception—the ability to sense where your body is in space. Warrior III also engages the shoulder muscles and challenges our focus, requiring us to connect with our breath and a focal point in order to maintain our balance.

The Practice Begin in crescent lunge (see page 50), with your right foot forward and your hands on your hips.

Find a focal point on the floor in front of you. Begin to lean forward and bring your weight into your right foot. Keep your right knee softly bent as you float your left foot away from the floor. Find your balance here.

Then, see if you can straighten your right leg, and continue to bring your torso toward parallel to the floor. Reach forward through the crown of your head, lengthening your spine to counterbalance your left leg as it extends straight back behind you. Gaze down toward the floor or slightly ahead.

Aim to level your hips as best as you can so that they're facing the floor. Roll your left inner thigh up, and flex your left foot so that your left toes are pointing down toward the floor. Draw your right outer hip back.

Keep your hands on your hips until you feel balanced. If or when you feel ready, you can reach your arms out to the side or out in front of you. You can also bring your hands to prayer at your chest.

Aim to stay three to five breaths. To come out, bend your right knee and step back into crescent lunge. See if you can exit the pose with just as much control as you used to enter it. Then change sides.

TIP If balance is difficult, stand near a wall so that you know it's there to hold on to if needed. You can also bring your fingertips to the floor or blocks to help you balance.

VARIATION 1: WITH FOOT ON THE WALL AND HANDS ON BLOCKS

In this variation the wall does more than help with balance; pushing your foot into the wall can help you find more length through your spine and maybe even a greater sense of power in warrior III. And because you're pretty much perpendicular to the wall, placing blocks under your hands can make the pose more accessible, "bringing the floor to you" to support balance and help you maintain a long, neutral spine. If you tend to turn your lifted leg out in warrior II, the boundary of the wall can help you keep your back leg neutral.

The trickiest part is figuring out how close to the wall to set up. Give yourself time to play with your setup so you find the perfect distance for you. Begin by measuring a leg's distance from the wall: Sit with your back against the wall and stretch your legs out in front of you. Note where your heels land and place your blocks—at their tallest setting to start—a couple of inches in front of your heels and shoulder-width apart.

Come up to standing with your toes a couple of inches behind your blocks. Come into a half-standing forward bend (*ardha uttanasana*, sometimes referred to as "half-way lift" or "flat back") with your hands or fingertips on blocks and your shoulders stacked over your wrists. Reach back through your hips and forward through your

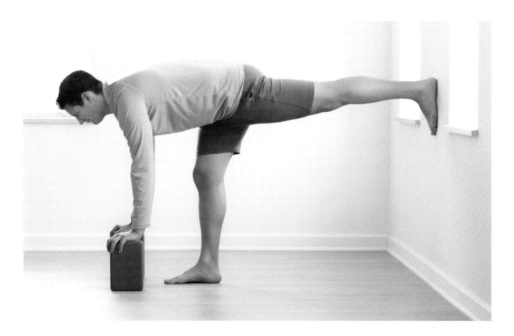

crown, lengthening your spine, bending your knees a little or a lot. If the blocks are too low, causing your spine to round, you can use a higher support like a chair seat. Or, if you can maintain your long neutral spine with your blocks at a lower height, feel free to lower them.

From here, stretch your left leg straight back behind you, bringing your left foot to the wall with your left heel at about hip height. You want the entire sole of your left foot, including the heel, touching the wall, your right hip stacked directly over your right heel, and your shoulders right over your wrists. To find this alignment, you might need to come out of the pose and move closer to or farther from the wall.

Once you're set up, check to make sure that all of your left toes are pointing toward the floor.

Bend your right knee to start, aligning your kneecap with the center of your right foot. You can keep the knee bent or begin to straighten it, drawing your right outer hip back as you do. Push your left foot into the wall and your right foot into the floor, finding even more length through your spine.

If you like, you can experiment with lifting your hands away from the blocks. Stay for three to five breaths, then change sides.

VARIATION 2: WITH HANDS ON THE WALL

For this warrior III variation, you'll begin facing a wall. Place your hands on it at shoulder height to begin (you may need to adjust a little as you go) and shoulder distance apart. Your palms can be flat on the wall, or you can come up onto your fingertips to challenge your balance more.

Walk your feet back until your torso is parallel with the floor and your hips are right over your heels, adjusting your hand placement as needed.

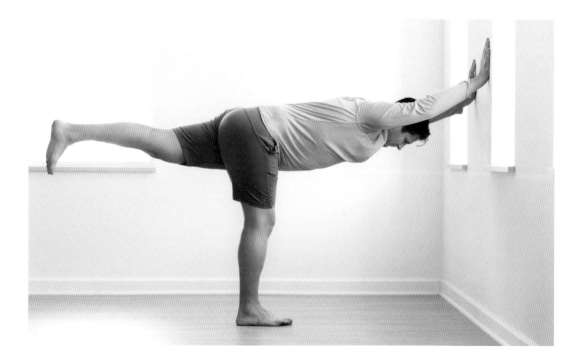

Press into the wall and shift weight into your right foot as you extend your left leg behind you. Keep your outer left hip rolling down as you spiral your inner thigh up. Reach back through your left inner heel and forward through the crown of your head as you gaze down toward the floor.

Stay for three to five breaths, then lower your left foot to meet your right. You can change sides right away, or walk your feet in toward the wall and your hands up the wall to come out of the pose, returning to standing so that you can take a break between sides.

TIP Because your torso is completely parallel with the ground, this variation requires a lot of back strength. To lessen the work in your back muscles, lower your back leg to a chair or block and/or walk your hands up higher on the wall so that your torso is at more of an angle.

VARIATION 3: WITH A STRAP

Similar to variation 1, this version of warrior III gives you something to push your foot into, helping you to find more length through your spine. The difference is this one provides more balance challenge.

Begin in mountain pose. Hold one end of the strap in each hand, arms alongside you, and step your left foot onto the center of the strap, so that the strap is in front of your left heel. Step your right foot forward, in front of the strap. Keeping your arms alongside your body, adjust your grip on the strap so that when you pull up on it, it feels taut. Lengthen your spine and begin to hinge forward at your hips, reaching your left leg behind you to come into warrior III.

Simultaneously pull on the strap with your hands as you push your left heel back against it. Stay for three to five breaths, then try the other side.

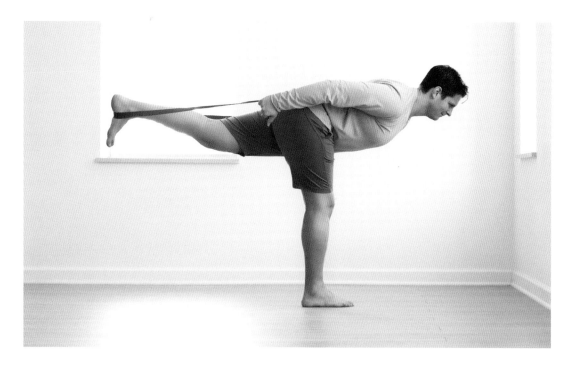

GODDESS POSE (Utkata Konasana)

This pose is also referred to as "goddess squat," "horse pose," and "fierce angle pose" (its intensity and power are what make it fierce!). Though this is a challenging pose to hold, it can be made accessible for almost all yoga students in one form or another.

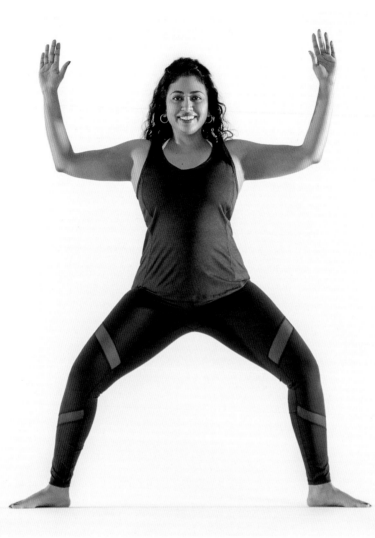

Benefits Goddess pose engages the muscles of the lower body. You might particularly feel your glutes and thighs working! Holding it for a set time (such as thirty seconds) is a great way to build strength and endurance.

The Practice Step your feet wide apart, facing the long edge of your mat, and float your arms out into a T. Make sure your wrists and ankles are aligned.

Turn your feet out, and come into a squat, keeping your knees pointing in the same direction as your toes. Bend your elbows to bring your arms into a cactus or goalpost shape. Stay for three to five breaths (or longer if you like!).

VARIATION 1: IN A CHAIR

You'll want to use a chair with a lower back for this one (such as a folding chair). Sit facing the back of the chair. Place your feet wide on either side of the seat, creating the goddess shape, so that you're squatting on the chair seat. Rest your elbows on the back of the chair, bring your wrists together, open your hands, and rest your chin in your palms.

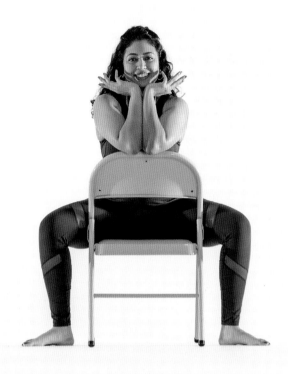

VARIATION 2: HOVERING GODDESS

Straddle a chair facing the back with your feet separated wide on either side of the seat, creating the goddess shape while hovering over the seat of the chair. Press down through your feet to ground yourself. Rest your hands on the back of the chair.

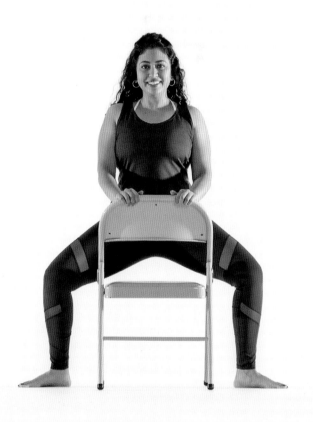

EXTENDED SIDE-ANGLE POSE (Utthita Parsvakonasana)

Utthita parsvakonasana (extended side-angle pose, often simply shortened to *parsvakonasana* or side angle) is a pose that often shows up in standing sequences. There are many different ways to play with this posture so that it fits the theme of your sequence (hip opening, chest opening, side stretching, core strengthening, etc.). Side angle also serves as excellent preparation for lots of other yoga poses. If you could pick only one pose to use as a warm-up, side angle would be an excellent choice!

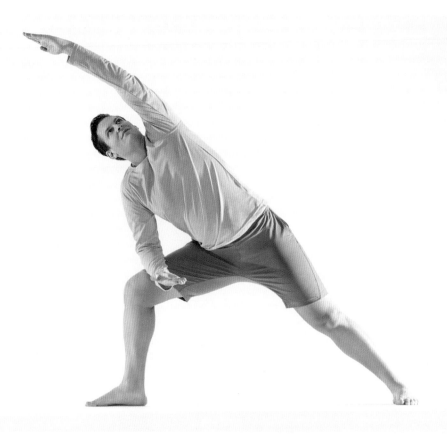

Benefits Side angle stretches the inner thighs of both legs, engages the quadriceps of the front leg, stretches the side body (in particular the intercostal muscles, obliques, and quadratus lumborum of the lifted-arm side of the body—the side that's on top), and activates the obliques on the other side (particularly in the "unsupported" variation).

The Practice Set up as you would for warrior II (page 72) facing one of the long edges of your mat, feet wide apart.

Turn your right toes out so they're facing the short edge of your mat. Place the outer edge of your left foot parallel with the short edges of your mat, or turn your left toes in slightly. Adjust your stance as needed so you feel stable. Bend your right knee, stacking it above your right ankle. As in warrior II, align your right knee with the center of your right ankle.

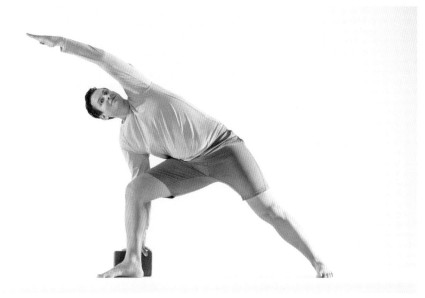

Bring your right forearm onto your right thigh with your palm facing up. Keep your shoulder stacked over your elbow. Bring your left hand onto your left hip.

Press your feet apart from each other, as though you're trying to stretch your mat apart (this helps to distribute your weight more evenly between the front and back leg). Press your right forearm into your right thigh to lift up out of your shoulder joint (instead of collapsing into it).

Stay here, or reach your left arm straight up toward the ceiling, or stretch it alongside your left ear for the side stretch, spinning your left pinky down toward the floor to bring a little more ease into your left shoulder. You can gaze straight ahead, or turn your head to look up toward your left arm or hand, depending on what feels best for your neck. Spin your chest up toward the sky.

When the front forearm is on the thigh, this variation is often called *ardha parsvakonasana* or half side-angle pose.

Stay here, or, bring your right hand to the floor. You can also place a block inside or outside your right foot and place your right hand on the block. Stay three to five breaths. To come out of the pose, look forward. On an inhale, press your feet apart from each other and rise up into warrior II. Straighten your front leg and switch sides.

TIP Are you wondering about when you might want to bring your front hand to the outside of your foot and when you might want to bring it to the inside? Here are a couple of points to consider.

Bringing your hand to the floor or block placed outside of your foot can provide a more intense sensation. This is especially true when you press your front shin or knee against your bottom arm and encourage your knee to move toward the pinky-toe edge of your foot. From here, encourage your bottom shoulder to roll back (it often tends to round forward in this pose).

If you're preparing for bound poses and certain arm balances, it can be helpful to have the bottom hand on the inside of your front foot, as that's often the position you'll need to come into to prepare.

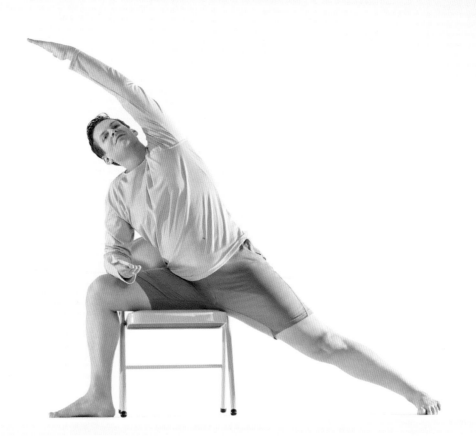

VARIATION 1: ON A CHAIR

A chair can make parsvakonasana feel more stable, which allows you to explore a greater range of motion.

Sit tall on the front of your chair. Widen your legs so that you are straddling the seat of the chair with your right hamstring supported firmly on the seat and your left leg extended out to the left. Arrange your feet in a warrior II position with your right toes pointing to the right and your left toes pointing straight ahead.

Bring your right forearm to your thigh, palm facing up, and reach your left arm straight up or alongside your ear. Gaze forward or up toward your left hand. Stay for three to five breaths, then switch sides.

VARIATION 2: HOVERING SIDE ANGLE

Want to make this pose more of a core challenge (particularly for your obliques)? From ardha parsvakonasana, without changing anything else, reach your right (bottom) arm out on a diagonal. This requires you to *really* recruit your core muscles to maintain the shape of the pose. Keep the back of your head lined up with the back of your pelvis and your chest spinning up toward the sky (avoid rounding forward). Keep your front knee bending. Remember to breathe!

Hold for three to five breaths, or, for a fun challenge, try holding for time: thirty seconds to one minute is a good starting place. When you're finished, rise up to warrior II on an inhale, straighten your front leg, and change sides.

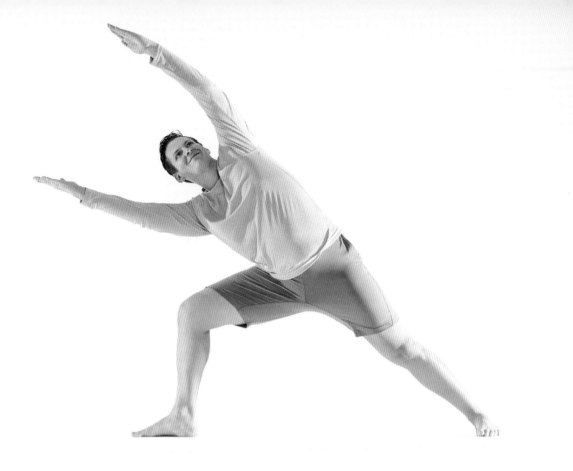

VARIATION 3: KNEELING SIDE ANGLE

If standing feels unstable and kneeling feels good for your knees (or if you just want to change things up) you can do any of the variations described here from a kneeling rather than a standing position.

Begin in a lunge, with your right foot forward and your fingertips on the floor on either side of your foot. Lower your back knee to the floor, toes tucked under. You can pad your back knee with a blanket if you like. From there, swivel your left toes to the right, bringing your left shin to a forty-five-degree angle. Lift your torso, turning to face the long edge of your mat for a kneeling warrior II. If you prefer, you can point your left toes all the way behind you, as Kyle is demonstrating in the photo. Find the position that feels best for your knee. From here, come into your side-angle variation of choice, and stay for three to five breaths before returning to a lunge and switching sides.

TIP This is a fun option to incorporate in a kneeling vinyasa flow sequence!

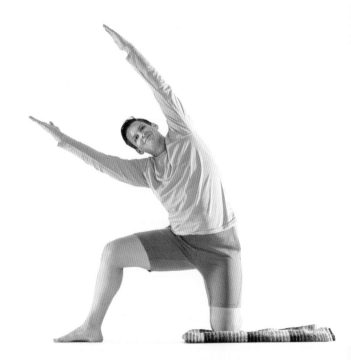

EXTENDED TRIANGLE POSE (Utthita Trikonasana)

Utthita trikonasana, often referred to as simply *trikonasana* or triangle pose, is a foundational standing pose, and a version of it can be found across nearly all styles of postural yoga. Nonetheless, triangle can be tricky to do. Its structure seems simple, but that simplicity is deceptive. This is a pose that requires a super-solid foundation, and a good amount of openness through your hamstrings. Here, we offer some suggestions that we hope will demystify and help you customize your triangle.

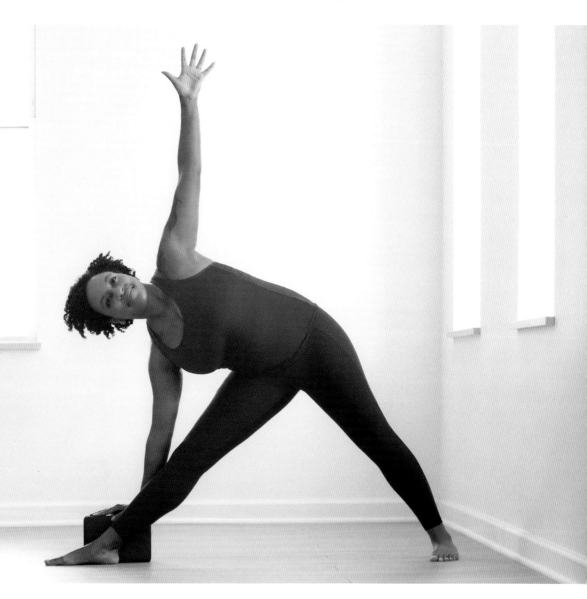

Benefits Triangle stretches and strengthens the legs and hips and opens the chest and shoulders. It also challenges and, when practiced regularly, can improve balance and stability.

The Practice There are many ways to approach triangle. While some schools of yoga teach triangle with a short stance, we prefer to practice it with a wide stance, with the feet as wide apart as they are in warrior II and extended side angle. Transitioning into triangle from warrior II or side angle works well for this approach because you don't need to change the position of your feet.

Begin in warrior II with your right foot forward and a block—at its tallest setting to start—behind your right shin. Straighten your front leg, but keep your arms in the T position. Adjust if needed so that your wrists are stacked over your ankles (or close to it—you're simply making sure that your stance is sufficiently wide).

Keep a micro-bend in your front knee and firm your legs by pressing down and out through your feet, like you're trying to stretch your mat apart. Keep your arms out wide in a T and reach out through your fingertips. Inhale here.

On your exhale, reach your right arm forward—to the right—and lower your right hand down onto the block, or your shin or ankle, whenever it can land comfortably without causing you to round your spine forward. You can move your block to a lower setting if that feels better.

Bring your top (left) hand to your hip, and stack your left shoulder over your right, opening your chest to the left. You can keep your hand on your hip or reach your left arm up toward the ceiling. Keep your gaze straight ahead or look up at your left fingertips.

Continue to engage your legs by pressing your feet down and wide. Stay for three to five breaths. To come out of the pose, look down toward your right foot, keep pressing your feet apart from each other, and on an inhale, rise to standing and change sides.

VARIATION 1: AT THE WALL WITH A CHAIR

A chair offers another option to create your custom triangle pose by using either the seat or the back of the chair to support your hand and bring the floor closer to you.

Stand with your back facing the wall. Set up in your wide triangle-pose stance, as described in the previous variation, with your right foot forward and your left (back) heel touching the wall. Place your chair against the wall in front of your right foot with the seat facing you. Stretch your arms out to a T, and inhale here. On your exhale, reach out to the right and place your right hand on the chair seat. Keep your left hand on your hip, or reach it up to the sky. Gaze straight ahead or up toward your left hand. Lean back into the support of the wall. Stay for three to five breaths, then, on an inhale, gaze toward your bottom hand, press your feet apart, and rise up to standing. Then change sides.

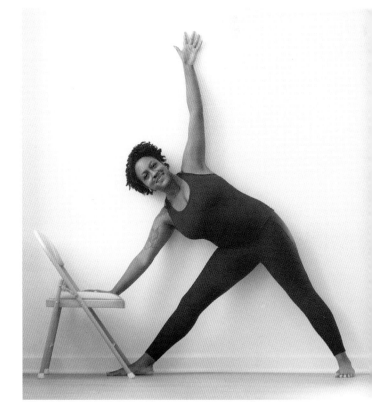

VARIATION 2: SIDE STRETCH AT THE WALL

This variation turns triangle into more of a side stretch, and the wall provides some additional feedback and support, allowing you to refine the lateral bend and to reap its benefits more fully.

Come to a wall (placing the short edge of your mat against the wall if using a mat) and bring the outer edge of your left foot against the wall. Step your right foot a little wider than a leg's length away from the wall. Turn your right toes to point to the right, and either line up your right heel with your left arch, line up your right heel with your left heel, or bring your right heel behind your left heel, whatever feels most stable for you.

Place a block, on its tallest setting to start, behind your right shin. Place your left fingertips on the wall at about shoulder height and stretch your right arm out to make a T. Inhale here, and as you exhale, reach your right hand out to the right; keep going until your left fingertips move away from the wall. Once they do, lower your right hand to your thigh, shin, the block, wherever it lands (note that it might be a little higher up than you're used to). Take another inhale here, then, on your exhale, reach your left arm alongside your ear, similar to how you would in extended side-angle pose (see page 82).

Spin your left pinky down to create more space through your neck and shoulders. Keep the back of your head lined up with the back of your pelvis, and spin your chest toward the sky. Gaze down, straight ahead, or up toward your left arm or hand. Notice if you feel a stretch along the left side of your body. To enhance that stretch, press your outer left foot against the wall and reach up and over to the right with your left hand. You may find that you'd like to lower your right hand closer to the floor, which is fine as long as it doesn't cause you to round forward.

Stay three to five breaths. To come out, on an inhale, push your left foot into the wall and press your feet apart from each other as you rise up. Switch sides.

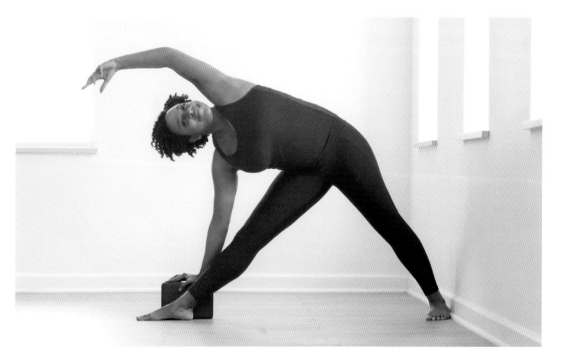

HALF MOON POSE (Ardha Chandrasana)

Half moon is one of our favorite standing balance poses—in part because you can transition into it (fairly) seamlessly from many other poses such as warrior II, triangle, side angle, and warrior III, and in part because you get to keep one hand on the floor! But don't let this asana's versatility (or that hand-to-floor contact) fool you: *ardha chandrasana* can be quite challenging for yogis of all levels. Still, we think the challenge is one worth undertaking!

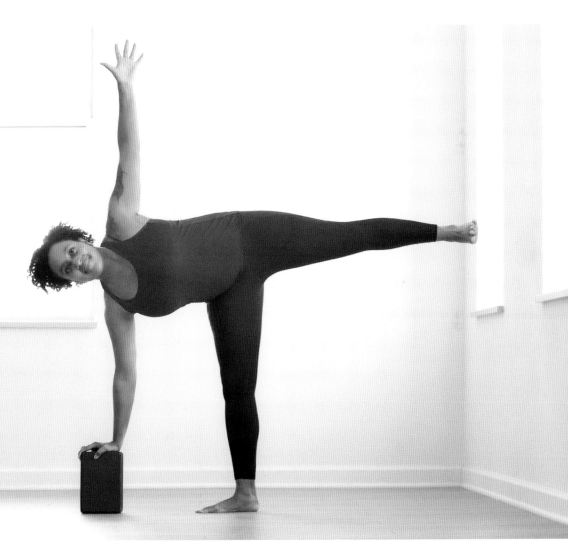

Benefits Practicing half moon regularly can enhance your balance and proprioception, and it also strengthens your legs, ankles, and feet.

The Practice Start in side angle pose (see page 82) with your right leg forward. Bring your left hand to your hip, and gaze toward your right big toe.

Keeping your right foot planted, step your left foot halfway forward and bring your right fingertips to the floor or a block six to ten inches in front of your outer right foot.

Shift more weight into your right foot as you float your left leg away from the floor, bringing it to about hip height.

When you come into the pose, keeping your right knee bent can be useful for helping you to align your front knee with the center of your right foot. With your right knee bent, you can root down into the ball of your right big toe and aim your right knee toward your pinky toe, which will engage the external rotators of your hip and prevent your right knee from dropping inward. Then, keeping that alignment, ground down through your right outer heel as you straighten your leg. When you start to feel wobbly, return your awareness to the points of contact between the floor and your standing foot—in particular the ball of your big toe and your outer heel.

Flex your left foot. Avoid swinging your lifted leg back behind you in half moon, which can throw off your balance. Either keep it in line with your lifted leg or bring it slightly forward, which can help with balance.

You can keep your left hand on your hip, or reach your left arm up, aiming to stack your shoulders and wrists and creating one long line through your arms.

Gaze down (best for establishing balance), forward, or up.

Stay three to five breaths, then see if you can exit the pose with just as much control as you had coming into it, gazing down, bending your front knee, and returning to side angle. Then switch sides.

VARIATION 1: BACK TO THE WALL

If you'd like extra balance support, practice half moon as described above but standing in front of a wall (with your back to the wall). This way you have something to catch you if you lose your balance. Be sure to leave a little space between your back and the wall.

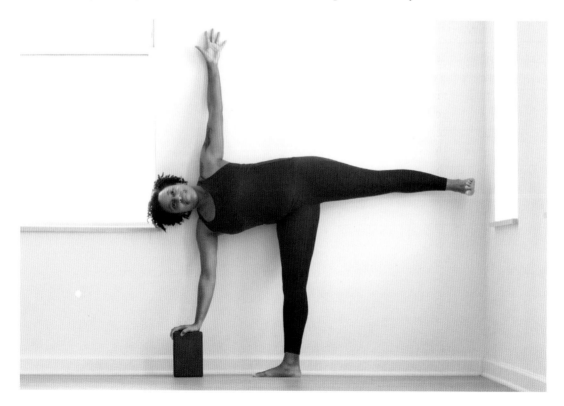

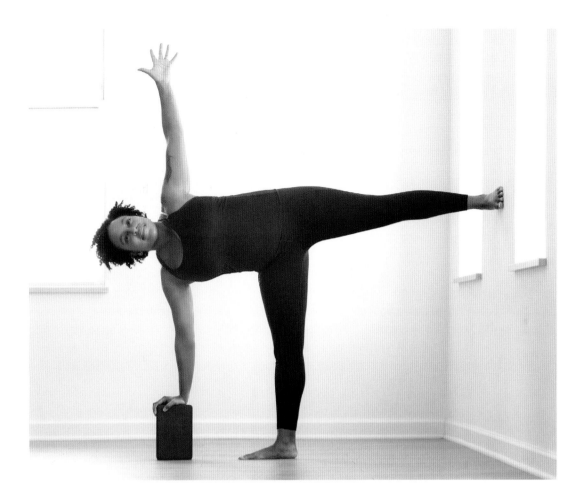

VARIATION 2: FOOT ON THE WALL

This version uses the wall for support in a different way, providing feedback to help you refine key ardha chandrasana actions. If you like to use a block in ardha chandrasana but find it makes you feel more wobbly in the pose, you might just find that pressing your back foot against the wall gives you the extra stability you need to *really* rock your half moon.

If using a mat, bring the short edge to the wall and have one or two blocks handy. Come into mountain pose a leg's length away from the wall, facing away from the wall. From there transition to *ardha uttanasana* (half forward bend) with your hands on your blocks on their tallest setting and your spine long.

Shift your weight into your right foot and stretch your left leg back behind you (as you would for warrior III; see page 76). Placing the entire sole of your left foot on the wall with your heel at about hip height (you may need to come out of the pose and move closer to or farther from the wall).

Lengthen through your spine. Adjust your block (or the block under your right hand if you're using two blocks) so that it's six to ten inches in front of your outer right foot. Then, without changing the position of your right leg, bring your left hand to your hip and open up into half moon, turning your left toes to face the left and keeping your left heel at hip level.

Press down into your right foot and resist it to the right—like you're trying to turn it out but can't, which will further activate your external hip rotators—and push your left foot into the wall. Stay three to five breaths.

To come out, return to your supported warrior III at the wall, step your left foot to meet your right, and then switch sides.

VARIATION 3: KNEELING HALF MOON AT THE WALL

(You can also explore kneeling half moon away from the wall.)

Begin in kneeling side plank (see page 178) near the wall with your right hand down and your left leg extended, the pinky-toe edge of your left foot against the wall. You may find it more comfortable to pad your right knee with a blanket.

From here, lift your left leg and plant the sole of your left foot on the wall, at hip height. You may need to adjust your distance from the wall. Make sure that your right shoulder is either directly over or slightly behind your right wrist—that is, that your shoulder isn't in *front* of your wrist. You can also place your right hand on a block (on its lowest, flattest setting). Keep your left hand on your hip or reach it up toward the sky. Gaze down toward your right hand, forward, or up toward your left hand. Press your right hand into the floor and push your left foot into the wall. Stay three to five breaths, then change sides.

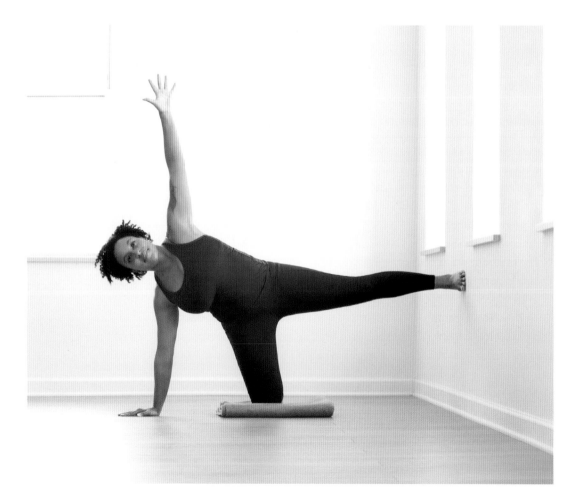

HALF MOON SUGARCANE BOW POSE
(Ardha Chandra Chapasana)

This half moon variation brings in a backbend and a sweet quad stretch. However, these added bonuses can make balance more challenging—but that's all part of the fun, right? Here are a few of our favorite variations to explore: whether you want to add more balance support so that you can truly savor the stretch, want some added assistance in catching hold of your foot or ankle, or simply want to experience the pose in new ways, we hope they inspire you to find an ardha chandra chapasana that's just right for you.

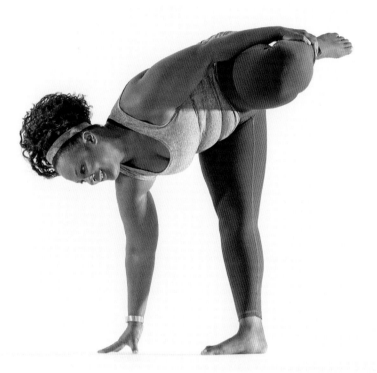

Benefits In addition to its balance-boosting benefits, ardha chandra chapasana stretches the quads and hip flexors of the lifted leg and opens the chest and fronts of the shoulders.

The Practice Begin in side angle pose (see page 82) with your right foot forward. Bring your left hand to your hip and look down toward your right foot. Keep your right foot planted as you step your left foot forward halfway and bring your right fingertips to the floor or a block six to ten inches in front of your outer right foot. Shift more weight into your right foot and lift your left leg away from the floor to come into half moon pose.

Keeping your gaze forward or down, bend your left knee in toward your chest, which will make it easier to catch hold of your left ankle or the top of your left foot

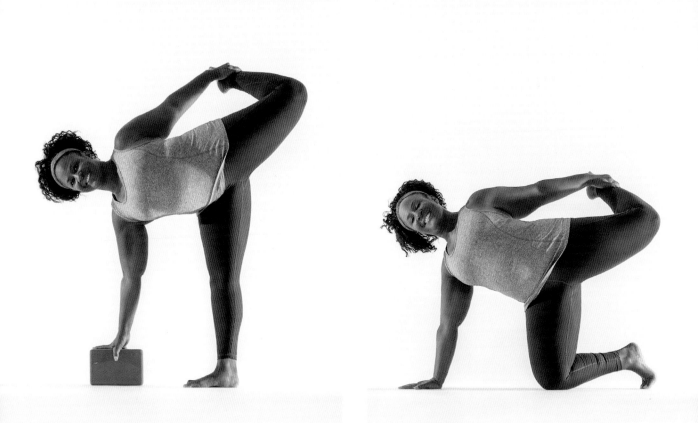

(or you can lasso your foot with a strap). This is a variation of sugarcane bow pose and a great place to stay.

If you'd like more of a backbend and quad stretch, draw your left leg behind you and press your left foot/ankle into your hand. Broaden through your chest and shoulders. You can continue to gaze down or forward or, if you feel stable, you might gaze up over your left shoulder. Stay three to five breaths.

When you come out of the pose, look toward your right foot. Aim to release your foot and step back into side angle with as much control as possible. Then switch sides.

VARIATION 1: KNEELING SUGARCANE BOW

This variation is great to include in a hands and knees flow or a side plank flow, and it's also closer to the ground, which can make balance less intimidating.

Set up in kneeling side plank (see page 178) with your right hand down and your left leg extended.

Float your left leg up to come into a kneeling half moon pose. Gaze down or forward and bend your left knee in toward your chest to catch hold of your left ankle or the top of your left foot. Stay here, or for more quad stretch and backbend, bring your left knee behind you, pressing your left foot/ankle into your left hand and opening through your chest and the fronts of your shoulders. Gaze down, forward, or up over your left shoulder. Stay three to five breaths, then aim to come out of the pose with as much control as you can. Switch sides.

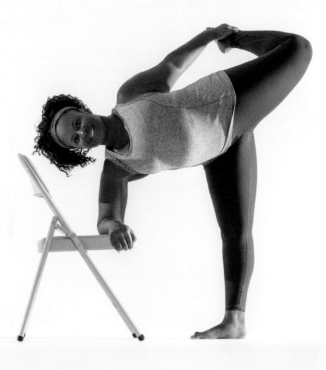

VARIATION 2: FOREARM ON A CHAIR

This variation offers balance support. Start by folding forward facing the seat of a chair. Place your hands on the seat. Make sure your feet are about a foot length or two from the base of the chair. Place your right forearm and palm on the chair for balance. Take your focus to the left, perhaps on the floor. Now, balancing on your right foot and right forearm, draw your left knee into your chest to catch hold of your left ankle or the top of your left foot. Press foot into hand and hand into foot.

Stay three to five breaths, then release and change sides.

STANDING BABY CRADLE POSE (Utthita Hindolasana)

This pose is a big hip opener that derives its name from the fact that you're cradling your leg as if holding a baby. Though it can be challenging, the act of cradling your own leg can remind you to be gentle and kind to yourself during this pose and all of your hip-opening practices.

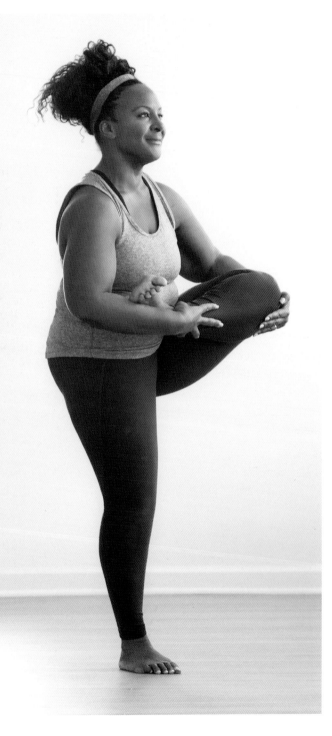

Benefits Standing baby cradle provides a big stretch for your outer thighs and glutes. It's excellent preparation for other hip-opening poses such as fire log (see page 104) and pigeon (see page 111), and arm balances such as flying pigeon (see page 189), which require a good amount of hip mobility.

The Practice Begin in mountain pose. Find a focal point on the floor, a few feet in front of you. Root down through your right foot and float your left foot away from the floor, drawing your left knee into your chest. Use your hands to draw the left knee close in toward you. Keep your spine tall and your right leg straight.

Then, bend your right knee, sit your hips back like chair pose, and cross your left ankle over your right thigh for a standing figure-four stretch. Flex your left foot strongly. Take a breath or two here. If this already feels like a big stretch for your right outer hip, you might stay here.

Otherwise, hold your left foot in your right hand, keeping your foot flexed and your ankle straight. Bring your left hand to your outer left knee or thigh and begin to straighten your right leg again, standing up tall, and lifting your left leg up, just as much as feels comfortable, perhaps bringing your shin roughly parallel with the floor. In this position, rock your bent leg from side to side a few times.

If you'd like to deepen the stretch, lean your torso forward to place your left knee into the crook of your bent left elbow and scoop your right arm around the sole of your left foot, bringing the foot into the crook of your right elbow. Clasp your hands in front of your leg and stand tall, drawing your left shin in toward you. You can rock your legs from side to side a few times here as well. Maintain your tall spine and stay for three to five breaths, then release your leg with control and change sides.

VARIATION 1: AT THE WALL

Using a wall or other support can help you maintain balance.

Start by standing in front of the wall, facing it, and come into the pose as described in the previous variation. The challenge will be to find the appropriate distance to stand from the wall and the appropriate spot on the wall (i.e., the appropriate height) to support your leg. Know that it will likely take a little trial and error. You can also use a table, chair, or countertop, resting your shin on top of it.

Once you have your bent, lifted leg parallel to the floor, rest your knee and toes against the wall, still holding your foot and your knee gently with your hands. Take three to five breaths here, then release and change sides.

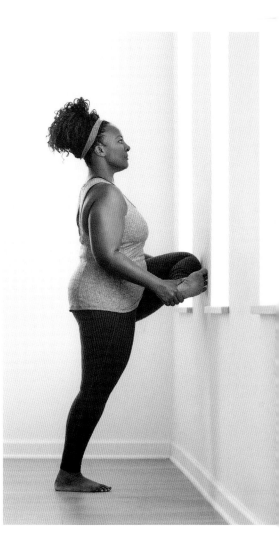

VARIATION 2: SEATED BABY CRADLE POSE

This variation removes the standing balance element altogether, allowing you to just focus on the hip stretch.

Sit tall with your legs out in front of you. If your lower back rounds, sit on a folded blanket or two to help you maintain a slight inward curve in your low back. You can keep your right leg long, or bend your right knee and bring your right heel toward your left hip (as Dianne is demonstrating in the photo).

Use your hands to draw your left knee in toward you, wrapping your hands around your left shin. Aim your left knee toward your left armpit and flex your left foot. Continue to sit tall. From here, hold on to the sole of your left foot with your right hand and bring your left hand to your left outer knee or thigh. Pause here and rock your leg from side to side a few times.

Stay here, or, bring your left knee into the crook of your left elbow. Either continue to hold your right foot in your right hand or bring your left foot into the crook of your right elbow. Lift your shin up, toward your breastbone, and sit as tall as you can. Rock your leg from side to side if you like. Enjoy three to five breaths here, then release and switch sides.

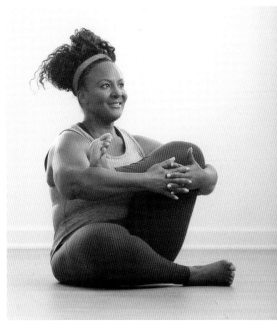

8

Hip Openers

BOUND ANGLE POSE (Baddha Konasana)

This seated hip opener is also referred to as "cobbler's pose" after the way cobblers in India traditionally sat on the ground to work on footwear. In Yin yoga, a similar shape is called "butterfly," and you'll often hear this name used interchangeably with *baddha konasana* as well.

Benefits Baddha konasana stretches the hips, groin, inner thighs, and back. It's an excellent preparatory pose for deeper hip-opening asanas.

The Practice Sit up tall on the floor, bend your knees, and bring the soles of your feet together. If your back rounds, sitting on a folded blanket, rolled-up mat, or block may be helpful. Press your fingertips or palms into the floor beside you and lengthen up through the crown of your head. You can stay here, or you can hold on to your shins or ankles, or use your hands to open your feet up like a book (separating the big-toe sides of the feet but keeping the pinky-toe sides together and on the floor) as you fold forward from your hip creases, maintaining a long spine. You can also rest your hands or forearms on the floor if that feels comfortable. Stay for several breaths. If you're in a forward fold, rise upright with a long spine when you're done.

TIP If you need to adjust the distance between your feet and your hips, try moving your hips toward or away from your feet instead of moving your feet toward or away from your hips. This can be more comfortable for your knees.

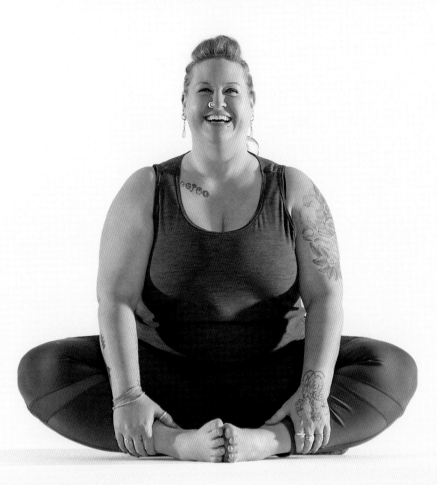

VARIATION 1: EXTENDED BOUND ANGLE (TARASANA OR "STAR POSE")

In this variation, the legs are less bent. You can think of it as a cross between *paschimot-tanasana* (seated forward fold, see page 132) and baddha konasana. If, like Kat, you're a fan of paschimottanasana but struggle with baddha konasana, chances are you'll like this wider version!

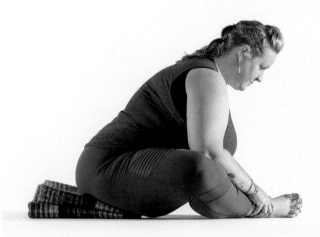

Set up just like you would for baddha kona-sana, but with your feet farther away from your groin. This position brings your knees down lower than they would be in a typical baddha konasana, which can make the pose feel more spacious and make forward bending a little eas-ier. As in the previous variation, you can hold your shins or ankles, use your hands to open your feet up like a book as you fold forward, or rest your hands or forearms on the floor. Stay for several breaths, then rise with a long spine.

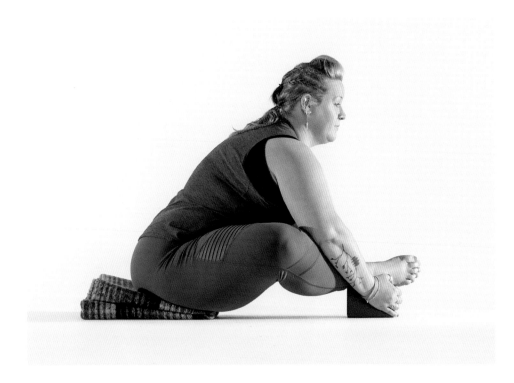

VARIATION 2: FEET ON A BLOCK

Often, those of us who find that our knees are significantly higher than our hips in baddha konasana (which can make it challenging to find length through the spine) are encouraged to sit up on the edge of a folded blanket. This is a great option for some, but if you tend toward an excessive anterior pelvic tilt (which just means your lower back curves in a lot), sitting on a folded blanket might encourage you to tilt your pelvis forward even more without making much of a difference elsewhere.

If that's the case, you might find it more helpful to elevate your *feet* instead of your seat, placing them on a yoga block on its lowest and flattest setting. Or, you might find that it feels best to sit on the edge of a folded blanket *and* place your feet on a block, as Page is demonstrating in the photo. Try all of the options and see which one feels best.

COW FACE POSE (Gomukhasana)

Cow face provides a great stretch for your hips and your shoulders at the same time. The shape of the pose is thought to resemble the face of a cow: The crossed legs create the cow's snout and mouth, and the arms form the ears. The torso creates the length of the cow's nose. (Look closely! Can you see it?)

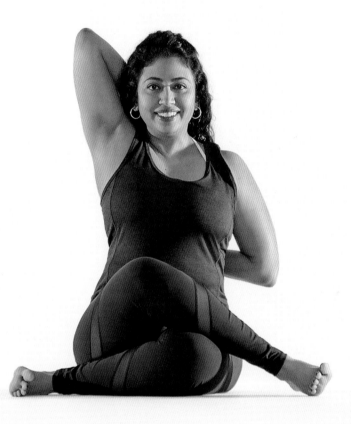

Benefits This pose targets almost every part of the body including the hips, shoulders, ankles, thighs, armpits, triceps, and chest. Working asymmetrically, as we do in *gomukhasana*, can help us to observe our bodies' asymmetries, noticing, for example, if the leg or arm position comes more easily on one side than the other. We can use this information to work with our posture and create a little more balance: perhaps starting on the side that feels more challenging or staying there for longer.

The Practice Sit on the floor with the soles of your feet flat on the floor. Slide your left leg under your right and bring your left heel to the outside of your right hip. Now bring your right foot around to the outside of your left hip. Try to stack your right knee over your left. Hug your knees together with your arms and shift your weight side to side, wiggling your hips until you are sitting as evenly as you can be on both sitting bones. If one side doesn't touch the floor, slide a blanket or two underneath your bottom until you feel supported on both sides.

Next, reach your right arm up toward the ceiling with your palm facing forward. Bend your right elbow and bring the back of your right hand to your upper back. Bend the left elbow and reach it behind you, bringing the back of your left hand to your back. Draw your shoulder blades together and try reaching for your left fingertips with your right fingers. You may need to wiggle and adjust to reach your fingertips closer together. It's okay if they don't actually connect. If the fingertips don't connect, try grabbing ahold of your shirt or holding onto a strap between your hands, as shown in variation 1. Lengthen your spine and actively reach your top elbow toward the ceiling. Try resting your head back onto your right arm to open your chest and bring your shoulder blades closer together on your back. Stay for several breaths, then unwind your arms and legs to change sides.

Note: Feel free to experiment with different arm/leg combinations. You can, for example, do gomukhasana with your right leg on top and left arm on top or with your right leg on top and right arm on top (and vice versa). See what feels best for you—just make sure to do both sides either way.

VARIATION 1: WITH A BLOCK AND A STRAP

The addition of a block and strap in gomukhasana can make the difference between a pose that feels awkward and a pose that feels awesome!

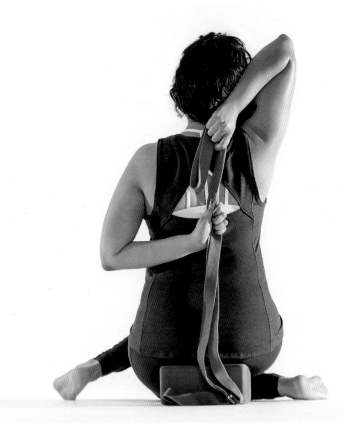

Begin on hands and knees with a block, on its lowest horizontal setting, on the floor behind you and a strap within reach. Cross your left knee behind the right with both knees resting on the floor and separate your feet so that you can sit your hips between them, onto the block. Using your hands for stability, lower your bottom to the block by walking your hands back and sitting down. Root down into the block and extend your spine upward.

Hold your strap in your right hand, reach your right arm up, and bend the elbow to bring the strap behind your back. Then bend your left elbow and reach your left arm behind your back to grab ahold of the strap. Walk your fingers together along the strap, until they're as close as they comfortably can be. Broaden your chest and lengthen your spine. After several breaths here, release and change sides.

VARIATION 2: SUPINE COW FACE POSE

If seated gomukhasana isn't working for you, or if you just want to experience the pose in a different way, try this supine variation. This version of the pose takes the arms out of the equation so that you can focus more on your lower body. If you like, you can come to a seated position and practice the arms on their own afterward.

Begin lying on your back with the soles of your feet on the floor. Cross your right thigh over your left, stacking your knees. Squeeze your knees together and bring your legs into your chest. Keeping your knees hugging together, grab hold of your ankles: left hand grasping ahold of the right ankle and right hand grasping ahold of the left ankle. Stay for several breaths, then release and change sides.

TIP To intensify the stretch, hold your ankles firmly and move your knees forward, away from your body, pressing your sitting bones into the floor. If grasping the ankles is unavailable try placing a strap across the tops of the ankles and using the strap to pull the ankles closer to your body.

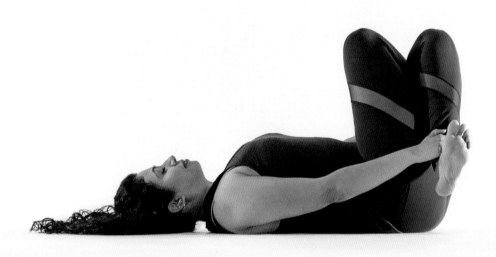

FIRE LOG POSE (Agnistambhasana)

Agnistambhasana (fire log pose) also goes by the names "double pigeon" and "square pose." It's an asana that calls for a good amount of external rotation in the hips. Generally speaking, if a pose like *virasana* (hero pose, see page 124), which requires a good amount of *internal* rotation, comes easily to you, fire log might pose more of a challenge. But don't worry! We have a few tips and prop hacks to share with you that just might make your fire log pose feel a little cozier.

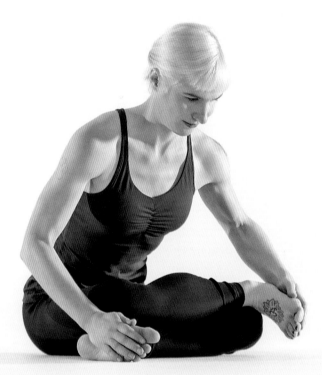

Benefits Fire log can provide a nice stretch for the outer hips, and may feel particularly nice after a run, hike, or a long day of sitting. And if you fold forward in the pose, it can provide a sweet stretch for your lower back as well.

The Practice Begin sitting tall on the floor. (As with most seated poses, if your lower back rounds, sitting on the edge of a folded blanket or two can help you to maintain a neutral spine where you lower back curves in slightly.)

Bend your left knee and, with your left foot flexed, arrange your left shin so that it's roughly parallel to the top edge of your mat (i.e., bent at about a ninety-degree angle). Then bend your right knee and stack your right shin on top of your left, right foot flexed as well, so that your right ankle is on top of your left knee and your right foot is off of your thigh. Stacking your right ankle (as opposed to your right foot) over your left knee might make your knee lift up a little higher, which is okay. This foot position can prevent your ankle from sickling (collapsing outward), which may help you experience a more satisfying stretch. You might find that placing your hands on the soles of your feet helps to keep them flexed, further helping your ankles to remain in a straight, neutral position.

Either remain upright or fold forward.

Stay for a few breaths (longer if you'd like!) and then come upright if you were folding forward and switch sides. For an interesting challenge, try to uncross your legs without using your hands!

TIP If your right (top) knee is a higher than you'd like, try this: While sitting upright in fire log, rock onto your right side, bringing your right hand to the ground as support; your left hip will be lifted off the floor. Bring your left hand to your left inner thigh and push the "meat" of your thigh off to the left (think internal rotation). Keep this rotation as you lower your left hip to the ground. You might discover that your right knee is lower than it was before!

VARIATION 1: EASY SEAT WITH FLEXED FEET

If your hips are feeling tight, *sukhasana* (easy seated pose, also known as "criss-cross applesauce" among the preschool set), with or without a forward fold, may provide just the stretch you're looking for, and it can be an excellent alternative to fire log. To make it a little more active, and to head in the direction of fire log, flex your feet and bring them a little more forward, aiming to bring your shins closer to parallel with the top edge of your mat. Stay for several breaths, and make sure to do both sides.

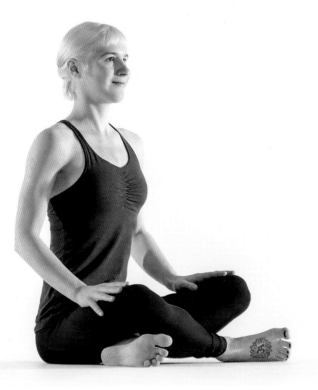

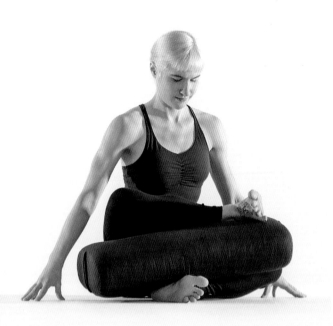

VARIATION 2: WITH A PROP BETWEEN YOUR SHINS

If your knees feel fine, but there's a lot of space between your top and bottom shin, it might feel good to fill that space with a prop, such as a bolster, block, or blanket. Experiment with different props and configurations to find what works best for you.

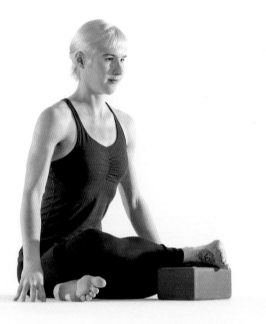

VARIATION 3: FOOT ON A BLOCK

If there's a lot of space between your shins and placing a prop under your top shin doesn't feel helpful, try placing a block in front of your bottom shin and resting your top foot or ankle on the block.

LUNGE WITH THIGH STRETCH (King Arthur Pose)

King Arthur pose is excellent for stretching the quads and hip flexors. Much like King Arthur in those legendary tales, this pose is intense! It can be a test for your breath and endurance, particularly if your quads and hip flexors feel tight.

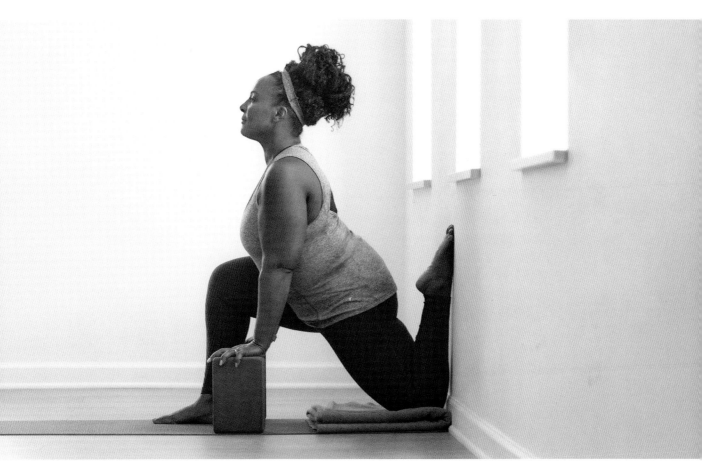

Benefits While a traditional low lunge such as *anjaneyasana* (see page 52) provides a quad stretch for the back leg, it only stretches the rectus femoris (that's the quadriceps muscle that crosses both the hip joint and the knee joint). If you want to stretch the other three quadriceps muscles (the vastus lateralis, vastus medialis, and vastus intermedius muscles, which only cross the knee joint), you have to bend your back knee and draw your back heel in toward your seat, as you do in King Arthur pose! It also is a great stretch for the psoas. Stretching these muscles is particularly helpful for backbend poses.

The Practice Begin on hands and knees facing away from a wall, with your toes tucked under and the balls of your feet against the wall. It can be a good idea to have a folded blanket under your knees for padding. Placing blocks under your hands can make the pose easier to get into as well. Take your bent left knee to the base of the wall, where the wall meets the floor, and slide your left shin up the wall, with the shoelace side of your foot pressed into the wall.

Then, step your right foot forward into a lunge, with the knee stacked over the ankle (this is where blocks under hands come in handy; they give you more space to step through). If stepping your foot straight forward is difficult, try sweeping your right foot wide out to the side as you step forward and then scooching it between your hands/blocks.

Find a position that feels comfortable for your hands. Hands on blocks can make this pose more accessible, but you can also put your hands on your hips or your front thigh or raise your arms to the sky. Engage your pelvic floor and draw your lower belly in. Lengthen through your spine. Stay three to five breaths. To come out, either slide your back knee straight forward or your front knee straight back and return to hands and knees. (Avoid twisting your back knee out to the side when you come out.) Then switch sides.

VARIATION 1: ON A CHAIR

Another option for King Arthur Pose is to use a throne (also known as a chair). The chair may make the pose more accessible or more challenging, depending on how your hips feel. It adds the challenge of a one-legged balance to the pose.

Start in mountain pose facing away from the chair. Find your focal point and root down through your right foot. Bend your left knee and place it on the chair seat behind you. Rest the top of the foot on the back of the chair with the sole of the foot facing up. Adjust the stance of your right leg as needed so that you can bend your knee and

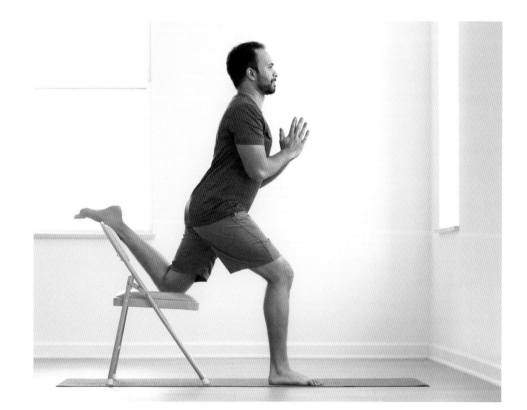

stack it over your ankle, making a lunge shape. Make sure you can still see your toes. Place your hands on your hips, on your front thigh, or bring hands to heart in prayer as shown. Engage your pelvic floor and draw your lower belly in. Stay for a few breaths, then step your left foot forward to meet your right, returning to mountain pose before switching sides.

VARIATION 2: LOW LUNGE WITH A THIGH STRETCH AWAY FROM THE WALL

You can also practice a lunge with a quad/hip flexor stretch away from the wall. This variation can feel less intense than King Arthur pose, but the trade-off is that it can be tricky to catch hold of your back foot.

Begin in a low lunge with your right foot forward and your left knee on the floor. From here, decide if you're going to:

1. Hold on to your left foot with your left hand (as pictured), or

2. Hold on to your left foot with your right hand, making this a twisted thigh-stretch lunge.

Some people find that one or the other provides a sweeter thigh stretch, so try both and see which one you prefer.

For version one, walk your hands up onto your right thigh. Press your palms into your thigh, and see if you notice a corresponding lift in your lower belly. See if you can keep that low belly engagement as you bend your left knee in toward your seat. Reach back with your left hand and catch hold of the big-toe side of your left foot with your

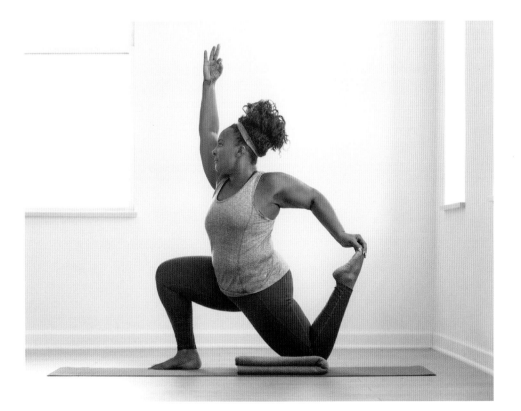

left hand. (Holding the big-toe side in this version can help to keep your left shoulder rolling back instead of forward.)

Keep your left toes active and lightly spreading. If you feel a big thigh stretch already, stay here. To deepen the thigh stretch, bend your left elbow and draw your heel closer to your seat. You can keep your right hand on your thigh, or reach it up toward the ceiling. Stay three to five breaths. When you release, instead of "sling-shotting" your foot, bring it back to the ground with as much control as you can. Switch sides.

If you'd like to try the twisted version, walk both hands to the inside of your right foot, moving it a little more to the right if needed. (It's okay to turn your right foot out here as well, but make sure your right knee and toes are pointing in the same direction.) Bring your right hand onto your right thigh. Lengthen your spine and keep that length as you twist to the right.

From this revolved low lunge, draw your left heel in toward your seat. Catch hold of the pinky-toe side of your left foot with your right hand. (In this variation, holding on to the pinky-toe side of the foot will help prevent your right shoulder from rolling forward.) You can keep your left fingertips on the floor or lower down to your left palm or forearm if that feels good. Keep your toes active, and if you'd like to deepen the stretch, bend your right elbow to draw your left heel in toward your glutes. As you breathe here, see if you can roll a little more onto the outer edge of your left knee (the back knee will tend to roll in).

When you're ready to come out, on an inhale, release your back foot with control and untwist. Switch sides.

TIP If you can almost catch hold of your back foot but not quite, try giving yourself a (literal!) leg up by elevating your back knee on a block. You can also use a strap to catch hold of your foot.

If you're working with the revolved variation and you get a charley horse when you try to catch hold of your foot, try elevating your bottom hand on a block (so you're starting up a little higher) before catching hold of your foot, and really take your time doing so.

ONE-LEGGED KING PIGEON POSE (Eka Pada Rajakapotasana)

Often referred to as simply "pigeon pose," *eka pada rajakapotasana* is probably one of the most familiar hip-opening yoga poses. It's not uncommon to see it offered as a deep hip stretch in classes besides yoga—dance classes, CrossFit, even on your bike in an indoor cycling class. But pigeon can be pretty polarizing: people tend to love it or hate it. For some, it's a sweet, feel-good stretch, while for others it's awkward, uncomfortable, or just too intense. We encourage you to explore the key elements of this pose in order to find a version that works for you.

Eka pada rajakapotasana can be practiced as a backbend, a forward bend, a twist, or with the spine upright. Here, we'll focus on upright and forward-folding variations in order to maximize pigeon's hip-opening qualities. For backbend and twist variations, see mermaid pose on page 154.

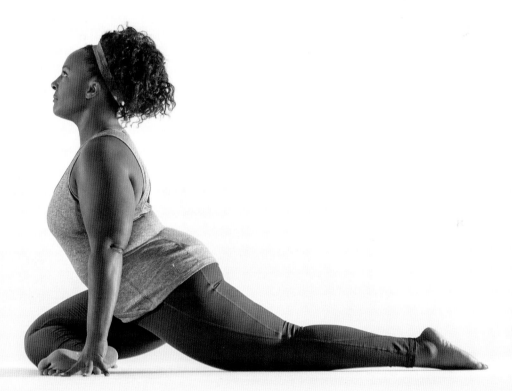

Benefits Many of us spend a lot of time sitting, which can lead to tight-feeling hips, as can activities like walking, running, and cycling. Pigeon can serve as a countermeasure as it's a great stretch for your hips and thighs, including the psoas, piriformis, tensor fasciae latae, and gluteus maximus.

The Practice From downward dog or hands and knees, bring your right shin forward so that your right knee is near your right wrist and your right ankle is near your left wrist (lower your back knee to the floor if you're coming into the pose from downward dog). Point your front foot but flex the toes back toward you so that your foot is in between flexed and pointed (sometimes called "flointed") and press the pinky-toe side of your foot into the floor so that your front ankle is straight, not sickled (i.e., not collapsing inward). Slide your left leg back a little, keeping your back toes tucked under to begin, back heel stacked over the ball of your back foot. Draw your right hip back and left hip forward until you feel the first sensation of stretch and stop there for now. Either keep your back toes tucked or point your back foot.

Walk your hands back toward your hips to come more upright, press your fingertips into the floor, and lengthen through your spine. You can remain upright or fold forward, perhaps bringing your forearms to the floor in front of you or stretching your arms straight ahead. You can rest your forehead on a block, a bolster, the floor, stacked fists, or wherever feel comfortable. Stay for several breaths, then bring your torso upright if you were in the fold and slide your front leg back to return to down-dog or all fours. Then switch sides.

TIP If you want to deepen the stretch, widen your front knee out to the side while you work toward moving your front shin more toward parallel to the front edge of your mat, and tuck your back toes (if they're not tucked already) and scoot your back leg back until you get to a place where you feel a bit more stretch in your front outer hip, and maybe the front of your back thigh too.

VARIATION 1: PIGEON WITH A BOLSTER

If your hips feel really tight, a bolster may help pigeon to feel better.

Place the bolster so that its long edge is parallel with the top of your mat. Then, from hands and knees or downward dog, bring your right leg over the bolster in a lunge position, with your left knee on the floor behind you. Now, heel-toe your right foot toward your left wrist, until your thigh and hip rest comfortably on the bolster. Press down into the bolster, supporting your right thigh and hip while extending your left leg behind you. Lengthen your spine. "Floint" your front foot, pushing out through the mound of the big toe. Your back toes can be tucked or pointed. Remain upright or fold forward. After several breaths, return to your starting position and switch sides.

TIP If you don't have a bolster, you can slide a block underneath your hip for support.

VARIATION 2: PIGEON ON A CHAIR

Using a chair and a bolster can both support and deepen your pigeon, bringing a whole new dimension to the stretch! This variation may be more accessible or it may be more intense depending on the tightness of your hips.

Start by standing, facing the seat of a chair, with a bolster in reach if you'd like to use one. Bring your right knee and shin to rest on the seat of the chair. Placing your hands on the back of the chair, square your torso to face the back of the chair. Scoot your left leg back and extend out through the heel. For more stretch in the quads and hip flexors of the back leg, lower your left knee to a bolster. Stay for several breaths, then switch sides.

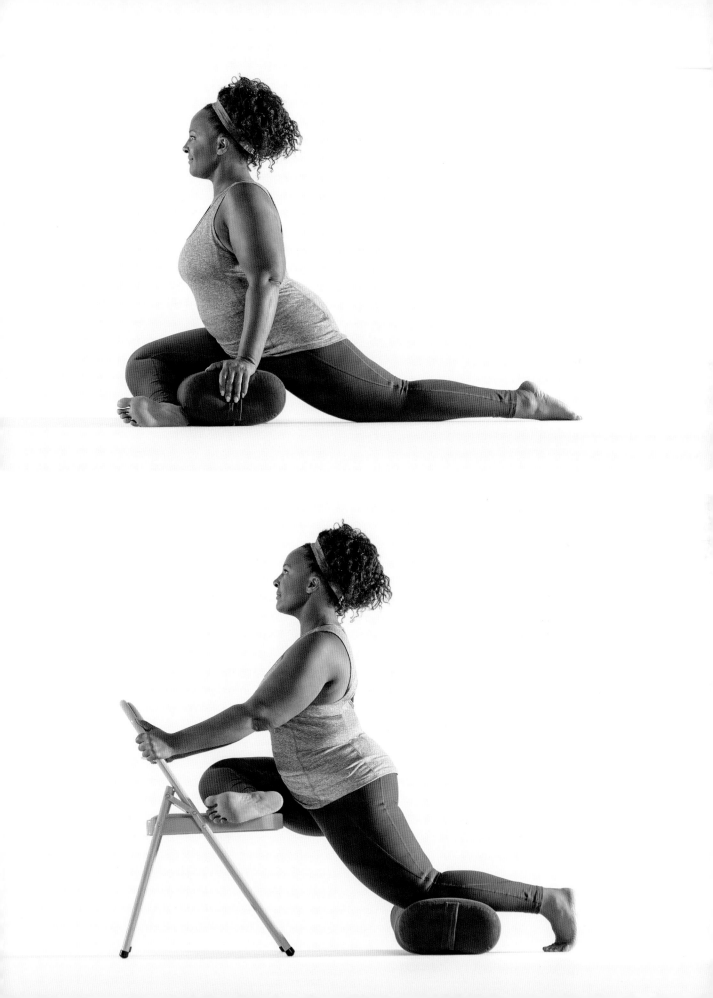

FROG POSE (Mandukasana)

This is one of those "love it, hate it, or *what*?" poses, meaning people either tend to see it as a feel-good stretch (love it!) or an *intense* not-so-feel-good stretch (hate it!) or they tend to not feel any stretch at all (huh?). Read on! We hope these variations offer subtle strengthening ways to explore the pose, even if you don't necessarily experience a deep stretch. And if not? Skip it! There are *plenty* of other poses to explore.

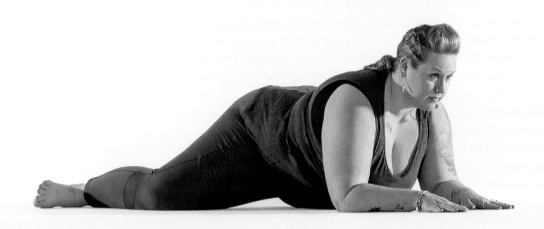

Benefits A favorite of many ballet dancers, frog pose can provide a great inner thigh/groin stretch.

The Practice From hands and knees, bring your big toes to touch and separate your knees wide apart—perhaps as wide as your mat. Sit back on your heels, walk your hands forward so your arms are extended in front of you, and rest your forehead on the mat. This is commonly known as a "wide child's pose," and it's your starting position for frog. Enjoy a few breaths here, then lift your hips so they're stacked right over your knees, and come up onto your forearms, stacking your shoulders over your elbows. Then, flex your feet and widen them out to the sides, away from each other so that your shins are parallel. Keep your spine long and neutral (maintain a little engagement in your lower belly to avoid overarching your lower back). Allow your legs to separate and your pelvis to lower toward the floor as much as feels good for you.

Stay for several breaths. To come out, walk up onto the palms of your hands, straightening your arms, walk your big toes back together, as they were in your wide child's pose, and then bring your knees together to come to a kneeling position.

VARIATION 1: PROPPED UP ON A BLOCK (OR BLOCKS)

Once you've come into frog pose, it might feel good to place a yoga block (horizontally, on its flattest setting or its second tallest setting) under your sternum, or your upper abdomen (between your navel and your sternum). Placing the block under your upper abdomen can be helpful if you tend to overarch your lower back because it can serve as a tangible reminder to draw your belly in for support (lifting it away from the block). You might also place a block under your forehead here. If you have two blocks, you could place one block (on its lowest, flattest setting) under each forearm. Experiment and see what propping feels best for you.

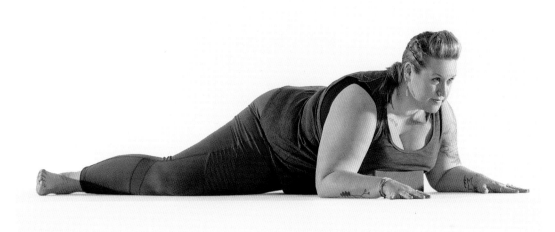

VARIATION 2: HALF FROG POSE (ARDHA MANDUKASANA)

If frog pose is too intense of an inner thigh/groin stretch, or otherwise doesn't feel awesome, half frog may be an excellent alternative. Set up as you would for frog, in a wide child's pose, and then lift your hips, stacking them over your knees. Keep your big toes touching or as close as they comfortably can be for this one and your upper body as it was in child's pose. Stay for several breaths, then return to child's pose and come upright from there when you're done.

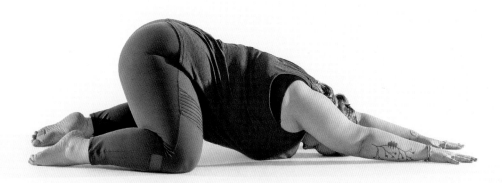

VARIATION 3: ONE-LEGGED FROG POSE (EKA PADA MANDUKASANA)

For this one, you'll begin in a crocodile pose variation (see page 211) lying on your belly with your forearms or palms stacked and your forehead resting on that stack. Keep your left leg long and neutral (not turning out or in) and bend your right knee out to the side in a frog position: knee stacked over ankle, foot flexed. Stay for several breaths, then return to your starting position and change sides.

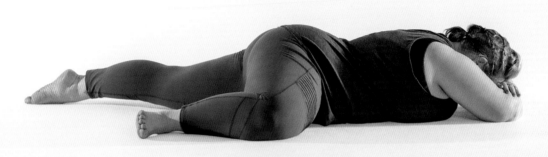

REVOLVED SUNDIAL POSE (Parivritta Surya Yantrasana)

Also known as "compass pose," revolved sundial is a fun, interesting shape to explore, but it can also be puzzling to figure out. The good news? There are LOTS of ways to approach revolved sundial and breaking down the pose step-by-step can make them easier to discover.

Benefits Revolved sundial pose is a great hip, hamstring, shoulder, and chest opener and it's wonderful preparation for the arm balance *visvamitrasana* (see page 179), which is also known as "flying compass pose." The complexity of revolved sundial reminds us that yoga is a journey and a process; it's not about "getting it right" but about getting to know yourself better so that you can figure out what works best for *you*.

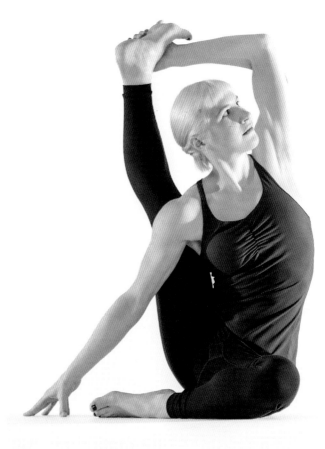

The Practice Start sitting tall on the ground with your legs extended in front of you. Bend your right knee and cross your right foot over your left thigh, bringing the sole of your foot onto the floor (like you might to set up for a seated twist), then bend your left knee and draw your left heel toward your outer right hip.

Think of this setup as the place from which you'll begin to explore any of the sundial pose variations.

From there, hold on to both sides of your right foot with your hands and lean back as you lift your foot up, which will help you to keep your spine long. Aim your right knee toward the outside of your right armpit to help facilitate the external rotation of your right hip. Bring your left hand to hold your right heel, and bring your right arm to the inside of your right leg and hold your right calf with your right hand. From here, we can explore our first question many of us have: *How do you get your leg back behind your arm?*

To "snuggle" your upper arm/shoulder under your leg, try lifting your right heel a little higher and moving your right thigh back to make space. From there, work your leg up over your shoulder and your shoulder under your leg. You can think of it as a three-step process: heel up, thigh back, shoulder under. Repeat this process until your leg is as high up on your arm as it comfortably can be. Once it is, squeeze your right shin against your right upper arm to keep your leg in place.

Next, let's look at two more common questions: *How do you hold on to your foot, and how do you work into the twist?*

Reach your left hand over the top of your right foot and hold on to the pinky-toe side. Now your head is framed by your right inner leg and your left upper arm. Bring your right fingertips to the ground and walk them out to the right so that your right arm becomes straight and you're leaning slightly to the left. From here, start to straighten your right leg (it doesn't need to straighten all the way).

Lengthen through your spine and spin-twist your belly and rib cage to the left; you're twisting away from your leg. Look down toward your right hand, or turn your head to look up under your left arm if that feels good. Stay for several breaths, then bend your right knee, unwind your leg and shoulder, and switch sides.

VARIATION 1: REVOLVED SUNDIAL WITH A STRAP

Practicing with a strap can make grabbing the lifted-leg foot more accessible, and it can also help you to sit up taller in the pose.

Set up just as you did in the previous variation, keeping a strap within reach. Once you've snuggled your right upper arm/shoulder under your leg and gotten your leg as high up on your arm as you can, loop your strap over the sole of your right foot and grab hold of it with your left hand—hold the strap as high up (i.e., as close to your right foot) as you comfortably can. Then, as in the previous variation, walk your fingertips out on the floor to the right until your right arm is straight. Then begin straightening your right leg as you lengthen your spine, twist to the left and bend your elbow out to the left. Gaze down toward your right fingertips or up under your left arm. Stay for several breaths, then switch sides.

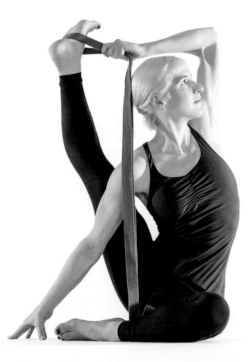

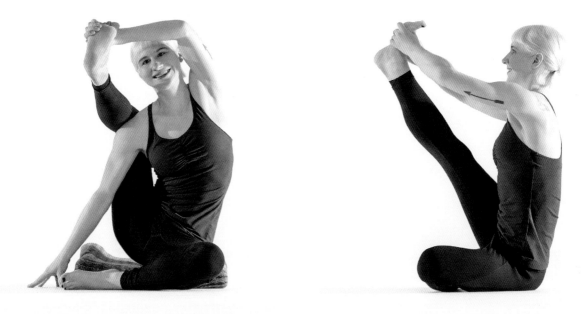

VARIATION 2: BENT-KNEE SUNDIAL

If it feels better for your hamstrings, or just in general, keep your lifted leg bent in sundial pose and your gaze straight ahead. You might also find that sitting on a folded blanket helps you to sit up a little taller.

VARIATION 3: HERON POSE (KROUNCHASANA) OR "UN-REVOLVED" SUNDIAL

This variation takes the leg-up-over-shoulder factor and the twist out of the equation, allowing you to focus primarily on finding length through both your extended leg and your spine.

Start with your same "home base" setup with your right leg crossed over your left and your left heel in toward your right hip.

Then, catch hold of both sides of your right foot with your hands (right hand holding the pinky-toe side and left hand holding the big-toe side of the foot). Lean back as you lift your right foot and bring your right shin parallel to the floor. Sit tall, lift through your chest, and reach up through the crown of your head. Keeping that length through your spine, start to straighten your right leg—a little or a lot, depending on what feels best in your body. Stay several breaths, then change sides.

9

Kneeling and Seated Poses

KNEELING TOE STRETCH

We're not gonna lie, this pose can feel pretty intense! But it's a great way to give the soles of your feet some love, whether you're a walker, runner, dancer, or climber, or you simply want to acknowledge and appreciate all of the amazing ways your feet move and support you throughout the day. And thankfully, there are many ways that you can customize this pose to dial the intensity up or down and find the perfect amount of stretch for *you*.

Benefits In case the name isn't already a giveaway, this pose provides a stretch for your toes and the soles of your feet, and it's a great way to strengthen your ankles!

The Practice Start kneeling with your legs as close together as they comfortably can be. Tuck your toes under, using your hands to help you (if possible, even try to tuck your pinky toes under, though note that this may not be possible depending on the shape of your feet, and that's okay—you're still going to get a great stretch). Sit back toward your heels. If your thighs are together, squeeze the inner edges of your feet—particularly your inner heels—together too. If there's space between your legs, aim to keep your heels stacked over the balls of your feet.

Sit as tall as you can, keeping in mind that the more of your weight that is over the balls of your feet, the more intense the stretch will be. This means leaning forward or back can de-intensify the stretch, so feel free to use this information however you like! Rest your hands on your thighs, close your eyes or keep them open and soft if you prefer, and breathe smoothly and evenly. Stay for five to ten breaths. Because this can feel intense, you may be tempted to breathe quickly to speed up the process. If that's the case, try setting a timer for a minute and remaining in the pose until it goes off.

VARIATION 1: HANDS ON BLOCKS

To make the stretch less intense, place your hands on blocks in front of you. This will shift weight away from the balls of your feet.

VARIATION 2: SITTING ON A BLOCK AND/OR PLACING A BLANKET UNDER YOUR KNEES

If your hips are hovering away from your heels, guess what? That's totally fine! But if you feel like that's not super comfortable, you might like to place a yoga block under your seat. Depending on your proportions, the block might be between your ankles or your calves. Either way, it can be helpful to squeeze the block to keep your heels from splaying.

If you'd like to give your knees extra cushioning, practice this pose on a folded blanket.

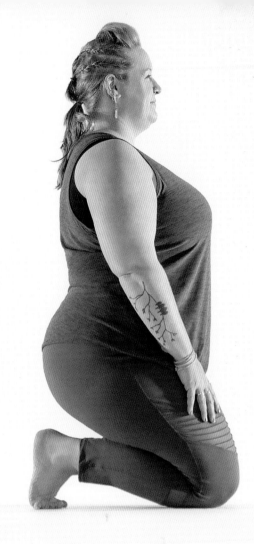

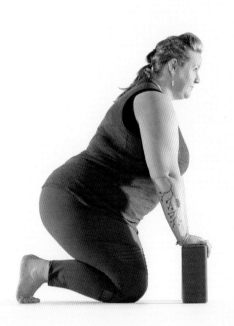

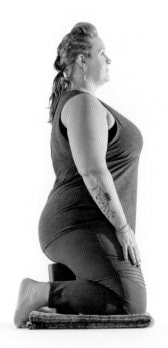

GATE POSE (Parighasana)

If you ask us, this unsung hero of side stretches doesn't show up in yoga classes as often as it should! Maybe that's because we typically don't spend as much time and attention on kneeling poses as we do standing and seated poses. Still, we think it's a great pose to explore, particularly because, as its name implies, gate pose can open us up to new potentials in our practice: as we make a little adjustment here or there, we learn what feels good and what doesn't, maybe even inventing new variations and discovering useful prop hacks along the way. Have fun with the suggestions we provide here, but don't be afraid to get creative too: this pose is all about opening up to possibility!

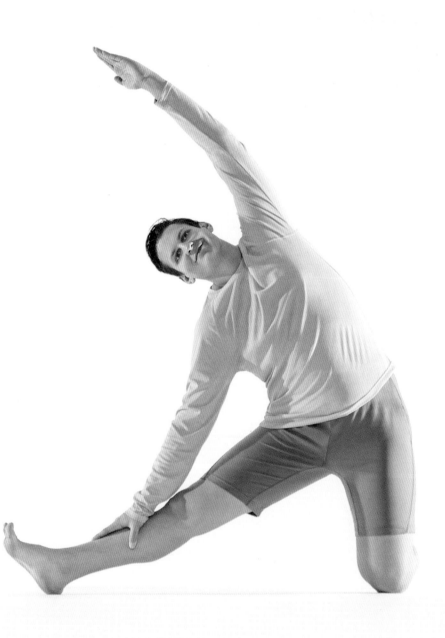

Benefits Gate pose provides a great stretch for the sides of the torso, and it also stretches your chest, shoulders, and the hamstrings of the straight leg.

The Practice Start in a high kneeling position with your spine long, hands on hips. Stretch your right leg straight out to the side. You can turn your right toes to point straight ahead and rest the sole of your foot on the floor, or you can keep your right toes pointing to the right, resting the sole of your foot on the floor, or you can flex your foot so your toes point up, as Kyle is showing in the photo.

Keep your left hip stacked over your knee. Your left toes can be tucked or pointed.

On an inhale, stretch your arms out to a T, and on an exhale, side bend to your right, resting your right hand on your thigh or shin (or a block in front of your thigh or shin if you prefer), and reach your left arm up and over to come into a side bend. Experiment with the hand placement that gives you the best-feeling side stretch. Avoid rounding forward, which will take you out of the side stretch. Spin your chest up, and find the head position that feels best for your neck, which could be gazing down toward the ground, straight ahead, or up toward your hand. Stay for three to five breaths, then, on an inhale, lift your torso upright and change sides.

VARIATION: WITH A BLOCK AND BLANKET

Kneeling on a blanket (or folding your yoga mat over for added cushioning) can help gate pose feel better for your knees. If you're working on ankle mobility and would eventually like to press the foot of your straight leg into the floor in gate pose, try placing a block under your foot. This gives you something to press into that's a little closer than the floor. The block can also help the pose to feel more supportive for some people.

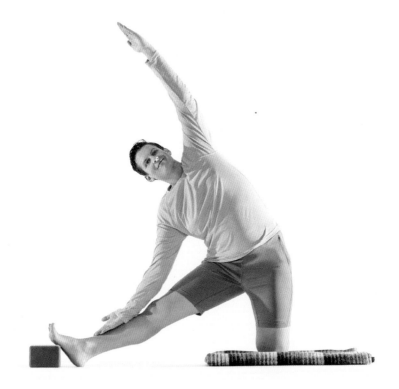

HERO POSE (Virasana)

For both of the writers of this book, hero pose doesn't come particularly easily; however, we still think it's worth exploring, which, as you may have guessed, means figuring out how to make it work for *us* instead of trying to conform our bodies to fit the pose.

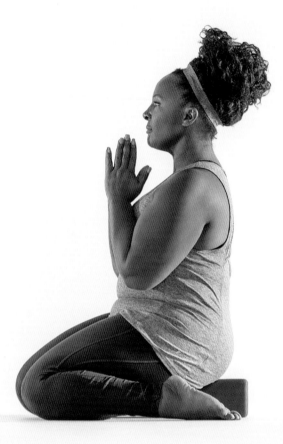

Benefits If your quadriceps feel tight, simply sitting in *virasana* might provide a nice-feeling stretch. It can be good preparation for backbending poses (many of which require pretty open quads!). Some people also find hero to be a steady, comfortable meditation seat, particularly when sitting on a block.

The Practice Start in a high kneeling position with your toes untucked. Separate your feet a little wider than your hips (wide enough that you can sit between your feet) and lower your seat toward the floor. You might find it helpful to use your thumbs to massage down your calves as you sit back, helping them to relax and maybe making it a bit easier to sit between your feet. If your seat is hovering far from the floor and/or virasana feels uncomfortable for your knees, place a block (or two stacked blocks) between your feet. The height and width of the block depend on what feels most comfortable and supportive to you.

Arrange your feet so that they're just outside your hips, the tops of your feet are pressing into the floor, and your toes are pointing straight back. If you're sitting on a block, hug into it with your feet and ankles to keep your feet from splaying.

Don't worry about having your thighs completely together in virasana. For many people, it feels better to allow some space between them. Sit tall, lining up the back of your head with the back of your pelvis. Rest your hands on your thighs, or bring them to prayer, or to any position that best serves you and your practice right now.

VARIATION: A ROLLED BLANKET FOR ANKLE SUPPORT

If virasana doesn't feel great for your feet and ankles, try placing a rolled-up blanket under your ankles for support. Even if you don't typically sit on a block in virasana, you may find when your ankles are elevated it feels better to have your seat elevated a bit too.

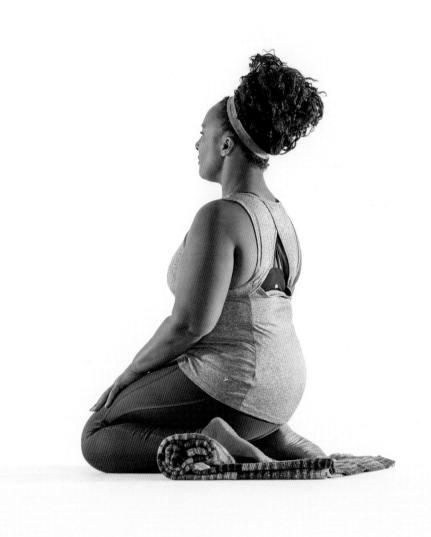

BOAT POSE (Navasana)

Boat pose is all about your core—and that doesn't just mean your abs. Though *navasana* is not an easy pose, we love how it makes us more aware of our posture and helps us to feel taller and stronger!

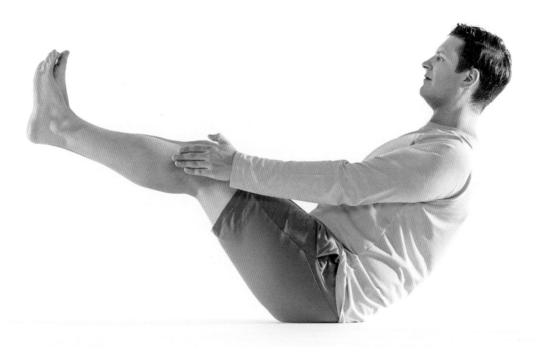

Benefits Navasana recruits and challenges the postural muscles of spine and abdomen, as well as the hip flexors.

The Practice Begin seated with your knees bent and feet flat on the floor, hands resting beside or behind your hips. Keeping your spine long, bring your awareness to your belly and draw your navel in on the exhalation. See if you can maintain some of that abdominal engagement as you inhale, finding even more length through your spine. On your exhales, see if you can maintain the length in your spine as you reestablish your abdominal engagement. Now, lean back slightly and lift your feet, bringing your shins parallel to the floor.

Keeping your core engaged, lift and broaden your chest, and lengthen the front of your torso. Then, extend your arms forward, in line with your shoulders with your palms facing each other. Stay here for a few breaths before straightening your legs to bring your body into a V shape. Stay for three to five breaths, then return your feet to the floor.

VARIATION 1: KNEES BENT, HANDS BEHIND THIGHS

For many—dare we say most—of us, practicing navasana with straight legs is extremely challenging (and honestly, counterproductive if it causes you to round your back). Instead of making straight legs the goal, aim to keep your spine as long as you can. Keeping your knees bent can help. You might also find it helps to hold on to the backs of your thighs. You can even use your hands to widen the space between your inner thighs, which can help to reestablish the inward curve of your lower back and allow for more lift and length through your torso.

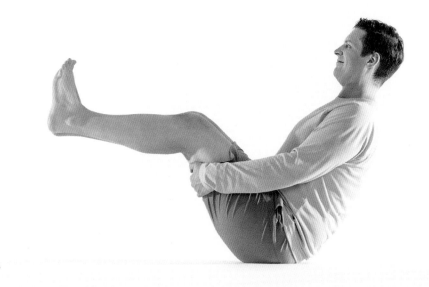

VARIATION 2: BOAT POSE WITH A CHAIR AND BLOCK

A more accessible option for boat pose is to use a chair and a block (or two blocks). Sit near the front of the chair seat with one or two blocks on the floor in front of you, on their flat horizontal settings. Place your heels on the block(s) and flex your feet. Lengthen through your spine, and hold on to the edges of the chair seat with both hands. Lean back until you feel your abs engage. Lengthen your spine and squeeze your shoulder blades together, opening your heart. From here, extend your arms out in front of you with palms facing each other. Stay three to five breaths. To release, hold on to the chair seat, place your feet on the floor, and return to sitting upright.

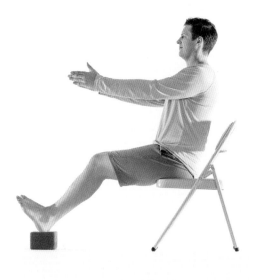

VARIATION 3: WRAPPED IN A STRAP

This variation can initially be tricky to figure out, but once you get your prop in place and find your "sweet spot" it can be super supportive and also pretty fun—your strap becomes your own personal, portable hammock.

Start by making a big loop with your strap. You may need to adjust the size of your loop along the way to accommodate your proportions. If you need a larger loop than the size of your strap allows, try linking two straps together.

Slip your loop over your head and bring the back of the loop against your shoulder blades. Make sure the buckle is within easy reach so you can adjust your strap if needed. Place the soles of your feet against the front of the loop, adjusting so that there's very little slack and you can straighten your legs (you don't have to straighten them all the way, though you can). Press your upper back and your feet into the strap—you'll find your "balance point" when both are pressing against the strap evenly. Reach your arms forward and lengthen your spine. Stay three to five breaths—longer if you like—then bend your knees, remove the strap, and lower your feet to the floor.

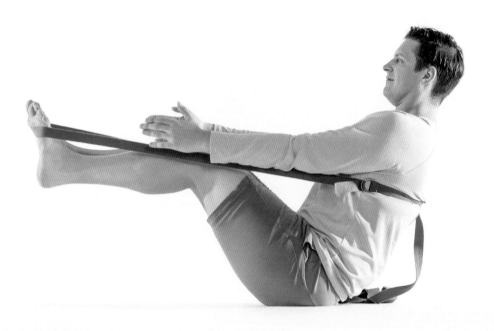

STAFF POSE (Dandasana)

At first glance, staff pose might not seem like anything special, but just as mountain pose is the foundation for all of our standing poses, *dandasana* is the foundation for all of our seated poses. It's where we establish a long, neutral spine to prepare for forward bending, twisting, side bending, backbending, wherever we're headed! But just as the pose itself can prepare you for numerous other asanas, it can be adapted in numerous ways to suit your needs and goals.

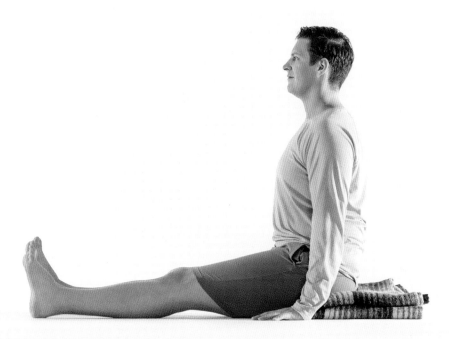

Benefits Dandasana is a great tool for working with posture from a seated position and helping you to establish a neutral spine. It can also provide a mild hamstring stretch (or possibly more than a mild one if yours are feeling tight).

The Practice Sit tall on the floor with your legs extended in front of you and as close together as they comfortably can be. Flex your feet. Lengthen through your spine, lining up the back of your skull with the back of your pelvis so your chin is parallel to the ground and your lower back curves in slightly.

If sitting tall is challenging or your lower back is rounding, try sitting on the edge of a folded blanket (or blankets), which can help to tip your pelvis forward and bring a slight curve into your lumbar spine. It can also be helpful to use your hands to inwardly rotate the flesh of your thighs (moving it down toward the ground and out to the sides) while still keeping your knees and toes pointing up to the ceiling.

Depending on your arm-to-torso-length ratio, you might be able to press your palms into the floor beside your hips. If not, you can press your fingertips into the floor instead, come up onto fists, or rest your hands on your thighs (while maintaining a tall spine).

VARIATION 1: LEANING BACK

This is a variation that we learned from fellow yoga teacher Amber Burke. It's great to try if your lower back rounds in dandasana and if sitting on a blanket doesn't feel helpful. Instead of trying to sit up straight with your spine perpendicular to the ground, walk your hands back behind you and lean back so you're at a diagonal with the floor. You might find it's easier to curve your lower back in here. Over time, you can experiment with walking your hands closer to your hips and coming more upright.

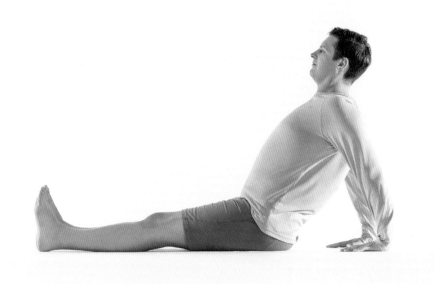

VARIATION 2: SUPINE WITH A STRAP

Like many seated poses, a great way to work with dandasana is to flip it upside down! *Supta dandasana* (staff pose on your back) takes gravity out of the equation: the floor helps you to maintain your neutral spine so that you can focus on other aspects of the pose, such as the hamstring stretch and the alignment of your feet.

Practicing with a strap can be an especially nice way to support your supta dandasana, holding you in the pose, and giving you something to press your feet up into. To begin, make a large loop with your yoga strap.

Sit on the floor with your legs extended out in front of you about hip-width apart, and place the loop over your head. Have the buckle of the strap in front so that you can easily adjust it if needed. Bring the back of the loop against the back of your pelvis and the front of the loop around the soles of your feet, moving the buckle off to the side a little so that it's not right *on* the soles of your feet. Then lie on your back, adjusting the strap as needed so that it's still across the back of your pelvis and not your lower back (it can tend to "ride up" as you lie back).

Press the soles of your feet up toward the ceiling, pushing up into the strap (it's okay to keep a slight bend in your knees if that feels better for your hamstrings). Tilt your pelvis forward slightly so that there's a little space between your low back and the floor. Aim to keep your chin in line with your forehead (if your neck feels uncomfortable, try placing a small pillow or folded blanket under your head).

Stay for several breaths. When you're ready to come out, bend your knees and allow the strap to fall off, then slide it out from under you and move it out of the way.

VARIATION 3: AT THE WALL WITH A ROLLED MAT

Like the supine strapped variation, practicing with your feet against the wall gives you something to push back into, which can help you keep your legs and feet in a neutral position. You might also find it useful to place a rolled-up yoga mat or blanket behind your knees. Why? For one, this helps you to maintain a slight bend in your knees, which may in turn make it easier to keep a slight curve in your lower back. Some people find it feels better for their hamstrings too, providing a less intense and/or more targeted stretch. It can also be useful if you tend to hyperextend your knees, lifting your heels away from the floor in dandansana.

TIP Note that for most people, there's nothing *wrong* with hyperextending the knees in a static, seated pose like dandasana, but keeping your heels grounded and pressing your knees into the mat or blanket roll can allow you to experience the pose in a new way.

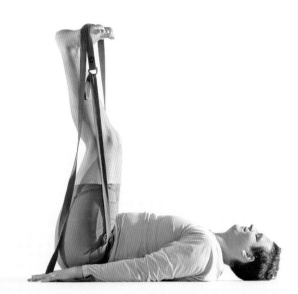

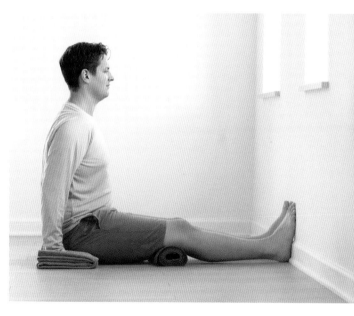

SEATED FORWARD FOLD (Paschimottanasana)

Paschimottanasana is commonly referred to as "seated forward fold," for obvious reasons, but in Sanskrit its name means "stretch of the west." Think of practicing toward the sunrise, greeting the day with a sun salutation, honoring the sun. The back of your body would, therefore, be the facing the west side, and in this pose, you're pretty much stretching the entire back (west) of the body.

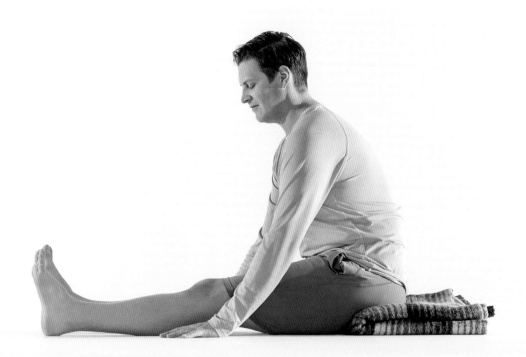

Benefits Seated forward fold stretches muscles of the spine, the backs of the shoulders, the back of the pelvis, and the hamstrings. It can also be calming to the nervous system.

The Practice As you set up for your forward fold in dandasana (see page 68) it's important to begin with a neutral spine. For most of us, this means sitting on the edge of a firm blanket (or two!) in order to maintain the natural inward curve of the lower back (otherwise the lower back tends to round, which can make folding forward difficult or uncomfortable).

Begin sitting upright with your legs extended in front of you and your arms alongside you.

On an inhale, lengthen up tall through your crown. On an exhale, hinge forward from your hip creases as you walk your hands forward, maintaining as much length through your spine as possible. As you release into the fold, you can rest your hands on the floor or hold on to your feet, ankles, or wherever feels comfortable. With each inhalation, lengthen the front of your torso a little more, perhaps even lifting out of the fold a bit. With each exhalation, fold a bit deeper. Keep your neck long and your face soft. Stay for several breaths, then return to an upright seat with a long spine.

VARIATION 1: BENT-KNEES PASCHIMOTTANASANA

If you feel restricted by tight hamstrings or your upper back rounds a lot when you attempt to hinge forward, try bending your knees enough so that you can comfortably hold the outer edges of your feet with your hands. You can also place a strap behind the soles of your feet and hold on to the ends of the strap as close to your feet as you comfortably can. This can take some of the "pull" out of your hamstrings and help you to maintain length through your spine and to achieve a more "evenly distributed" rounding as you fold, allowing more areas of your back to experience the stretch.

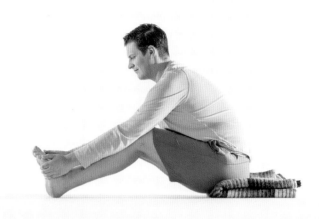

VARIATION 2: RECLINED PASCHIMOTTANASANA

Flipping this pose on its back can make it more accessible, particularly if the seated version of the pose doesn't feel good for your hamstrings or lower back.

Begin by lying on your back with your knees bent and feet on the floor. Rest your arms alongside you. If the back of your neck feels uncomfortable, place a folded blanket or pillow behind your head.

Draw one knee at a time into your abdomen. Once both knees are in toward your chest, stretch your legs to the sky, flexing your feet.

You can keep your arms alongside you or reach up and grab behind your thighs or calves or hold on to your feet. As long as it feels good in your body, your pelvis can lift away from the floor in order to bring your legs in closer toward you. Stay for several breaths, then return to your starting position.

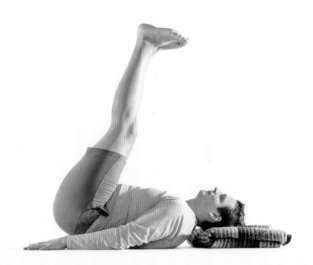

HEAD-TO-KNEE POSE (Janu Sirsanana)

Though *janu sirsasana* is often referred to as "head-to-knee pose," it's important to note that touching your head to your knee is not necessary and may not be available to you. That's why some teachers prefer to call it "head-of-the-knee pose," which refers to the common instruction to extend out through the head of your bent-leg knee while folding forward over your straight leg. Whatever you choose to call this asana, instead of aiming to touch your head to your straight-leg knee—or any particular place on your leg for that matter—focus on extending your torso long throughout the pose.

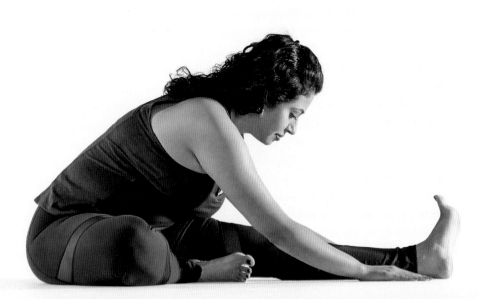

Benefits Janu sirsasana provides a deep stretch for your hamstrings, groin, hips, and back muscles. Forward folds can also feel calming and grounding for many people.

The Practice If your hips or lower back feel tight, sit on the edge of a firm blanket. If not, sit on your mat with your legs in front of you in staff pose (see page 129). Bring the sole of your right foot to the inside of your left thigh. Align your torso and collarbones with your left leg. Keeping your spine long, exhale as you bend forward over your left leg. Hold on to your left leg's shin, ankle, or foot. You can also wrap a strap around the sole of your left foot and hold it firmly with both hands. With each inhalation, lengthen the front of your torso. With each exhalation, fold deeper. Stay for several breaths, then, on an inhale, rise up with a long spine and change sides.

TIP Keeping the name "head-of-the-knee pose" in mind, you may find it useful to focus on extending out through your bent-leg knee while folding forward over your straight leg.

VARIATION 1: WITH A BOLSTER AND A CHAIR

Try this version if you'd like a more restorative experience, or if you'd like to practice the pose with less of a forward fold.

Place a bolster lengthwise on a chair seat and sit facing the chair seat, with your legs extended forward, in between the legs of the chair. Sit back far enough so that when you hinge forward your forehead will rest on the bolster. Keep your left leg straight and bend your right knee, bringing the sole of your right foot to your left inner thigh.

Inhale here, and as you exhale, begin to hinge forward slightly, maintaining a long spine. You can rest your forehead directly on the bolster, perhaps holding on to the legs of the chair or grasping either side of the chair above the seat. Or, for a little more height, you can stack your palms or forearms on top of each other and rest your forehead on that stack. If you'd like to add additional height you can stack a folded blanket on top of the bolster.

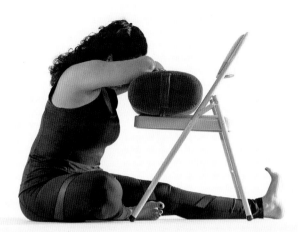

If you like the chair variation but want to deepen the forward fold, try scooting back (away from the chair) a little and using a lower support for your forehead, such as a folded blanket or two. Adjust as necessary so you can maintain length through your spine as you fold. Here too, place your hands wherever is comfortable.

Stay for several breaths, then, on an inhale, rise up with a long spine and change sides.

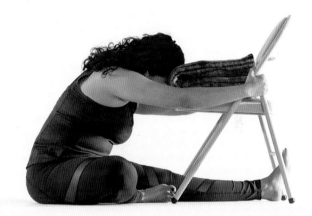

10

Backbends

RECLINED HERO POSE (Supta Virasana)

Like its upright companion virasana (see page 124), *supta virasana* can be challenging if the internal rotation of the thighs it requires doesn't come easily to you. Again, we cannot reiterate enough that this has nothing to do with your prowess as a yogi and everything to do with your hip structure, body proportions, and other anatomical factors—factors that likely put you at an advantage when it comes to other poses! And even if reclined hero doesn't ever feel "effortless," there are plenty of variations you can try to make it feel *good*—and, most important, to make it your *own*.

Benefits Even more than virasana, supta virasana is a great preparation for backbends like wheel, bow, and camel. That's because it provides not only a fabulous quad and hip-flexor stretch, but some nice chest and shoulder opening too.

The Practice Begin in a high kneeling position with toes untucked. Separate your feet wider than your hips so that you can sit between them, and lower your seat toward the floor (you can sit on a block or folded blanket if the floor feels far away). Arrange your feet so they're just outside your hips, the tops of your feet are pressing into the floor, and your toes are pointing straight back. If you're sitting on a prop, hug into it with your feet and ankles and reach back through your big toes. Take a few breaths to settle in.

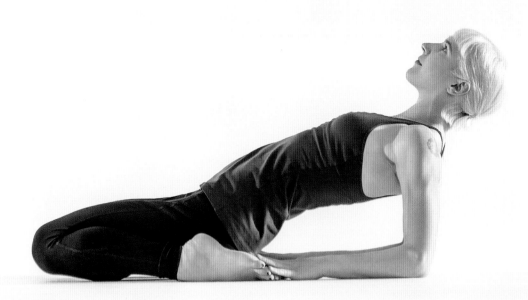

Once you feel comfortable, begin to recline back, first walking back onto your palms, resting your hands on the ground. (If you're sitting on a block, this is likely as far as you'll be able to go, unless you also have a bolster or a stack of blankets behind you to support your middle and upper back, neck, and head.) If that feels comfortable, you might come onto your elbows (as Kat is demonstrating in the photo) or even all the way onto your back—perhaps reaching your arms up overhead and resting the back of your hands on the floor. If you feel discomfort in your knees, that's a sign to back off and come more upright. Stay for several breaths, or as long as you like—perhaps even setting a timer for a minute or two. Press yourself upright and rise back up to high kneeling when you're done.

VARIATION 1: HALF SADDLE

If supta virasana feels uncomfortable, try half saddle. Begin in a "Z-sit," leaning onto your right hip and swinging your legs off to the left, bringing the sole of your right foot to rest against your left inner thigh, just below the left knee. Bring your left foot as close to your left outer hip as you comfortably can, with all of your left-foot toes pointing straight back.

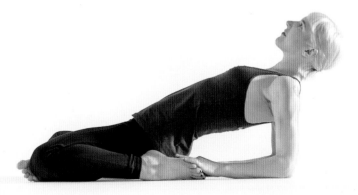

If this feels comfortable, you can start to lean back, placing your palms on the floor behind you, coming onto your forearms, or lying all the way back and placing your head on the floor (resting your hands in whatever position feels good).

VARIATION 2: BLOCK SUPPORTING THORACIC SPINE

If you can make it down onto your forearms in supta virasana, but lying on the floor is uncomfortable or out of reach, try placing a block behind your thoracic spine (middle back). The block can be on its lowest, medium, or tallest setting depending on what feels best for you. Some people like to have the block on its horizontal setting (the wide way), others prefer the vertical setting (the long way). Experiment and see what feels best. Whichever block orientation you go with, as a general starting point, line up the bottom edge of the block with the bottom tips of your shoulder blades. Gaze wherever is most comfortable for your neck. That might mean keeping your head in a neutral position or resting the back of your head on a second block, a bolster, a blanket, or even the floor if that's available to you.

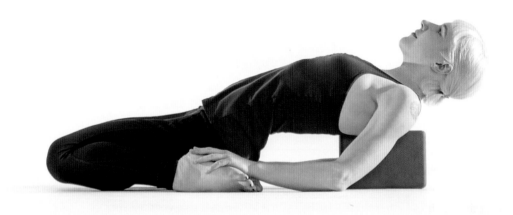

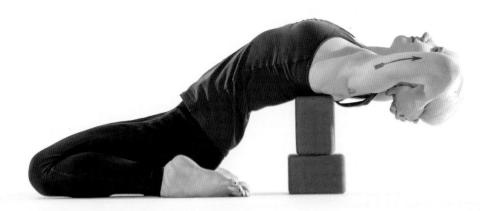

VARIATION 3: TWO BLOCKS SUPPORTING THE THORACIC SPINE AND HANDS BEHIND THE HEAD

This is the ultimate "lie back and relax" version of supta virasana! For this version, stack two blocks on top of each other: one on its lowest horizontal setting on the bottom and another on its medium horizontal setting on top. Arrange the blocks behind you so that when you lie back over them from your virasana position the bottom edge of the top block is underneath the bottom tips of your shoulder blades.

Remember, though, you're the architect of your practice: if this particular setup doesn't feel good for you, you can change up the position and orientation of the blocks until you find something that does feel good. Find a setup where your knees remain on the ground and you get a nice opening through your chest.

Interlace your hands behind your head and allow your head to rest back into the support of your hands. You might find that it feels nice for your neck to apply a bit of gentle traction with your hands, resisting them up toward your crown, but not actually moving them. Soften your face and jaw.

When you're ready to come upright, lead with your chest, as though your heart were being gently pulled forward by a string, and let your head come up last.

CAMEL POSE (Ustrasana)

Camel is often used as a preparatory pose for deeper backbends like wheel (see page 147), and is a great pose to do if you perform a lot of daily tasks that involve folding forward or sitting in a slouched or hunched position.

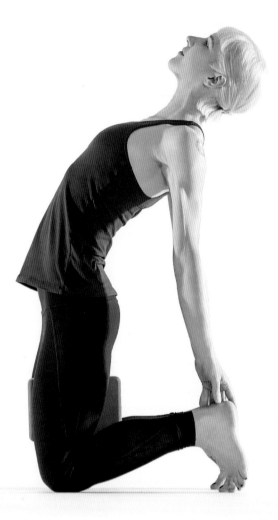

Benefits Camel stretches the front of the body including the quads, hip flexors, abdominals, chest, and the front of the neck and shoulders. It engages the back muscles and can aid in posture, and it can also have an overall energizing effect, helping us to feel vitalized and awake!

The Practice Begin in an upright kneeling position with your knees underneath your hips. (You can kneel on a blanket for added cushioning if you like.) We recommend placing a block between your upper inner thighs and squeezing it as you rotate your thighs inward and lightly engage your pelvic floor and low belly. This will help you keep your legs active and can prevent you from bringing the backbend primarily into your lower back, which is common.

Place your hands on your hips. Press your shins and the tops of your feet into the floor, or tuck your toes under to bring your heels closer to you. Rest your palms on the back of your pelvis at the bottom of your waist and the top of your glutes, with your fingers pointing toward the floor. Keep squeezing the block, lengthen your spine, and lean back, with your chin slightly tucked.

Stay here, or, if you want more sensation, reach back and hold your heels with your thumbs pointing out.

Make sure your hips are still directly over your knees. Continue to hug the block. Broaden your chest to bring the backbend more into your upper back. Gaze forward or toward the ceiling if that feels comfortable. Stay for three to five breaths.

To release, bring your hands back to your hips. On an inhale, lead with your heart to come up.

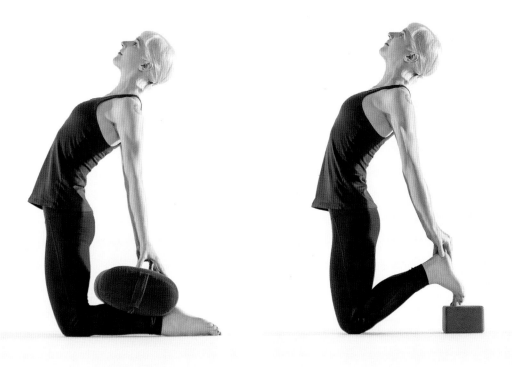

VARIATION 1: HANDS TO A BOLSTER

If your heels feel far away or reaching for them feels uncomfortable, you can place a bolster lengthwise across your calves and bring your fingertips to the bolster instead (if you need more height, place a folded blanket on top of the bolster). This is a particularly good variation to try if tucking your toes under is uncomfortable.

VARIATION 2: FEET ON A BLOCK

If you'd like to bring your hands to your heels, but can't *quite* reach them comfortably, try placing a block (on its lowest horizontal setting) under your toes for a little extra lift.

VARIATION 3: AT THE WALL

This variation is a great way to ensure your lower back isn't taking on the brunt of the backbend. If your thighs move away from the wall, you know you've gone too far. You can also combine it with the bolster and block variations if you like.

Come to a high kneeling position against a wall with your knees under your hips, toes tucked or pointed. Bring your hands to the back of your pelvis with your fingers pointing down. Lift your lower belly and lengthen up through the crown of your head. Then, keeping your thighs against the wall, peel your chest away from the wall, keeping it lifted and broad to bring more of the backbend into your upper back.

Stay here, or reach your hands to your heels, keeping your thighs against the wall. Keep your gaze toward the wall, or allow your head to move back into the arc of the backbend if that feels fine for your neck. Stay three to five breaths, then lead with your chest to come back to your starting position, letting your head come up last.

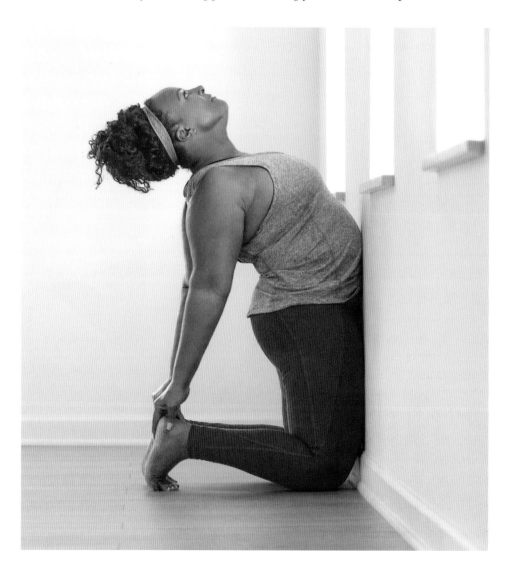

BOW POSE (Dhanurasana)

Bow pose is a downward-facing wheel pose that is weighted through your hips and thighs. *Dhanurasana* is a pose that's challenging for many of us, but there are several ways to make it more accessible.

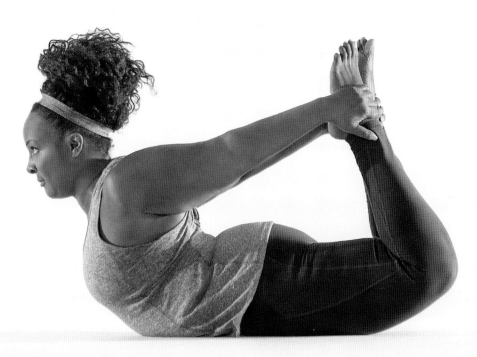

Benefits Bow opens the front of the body while engaging the back of the body. It stretches the chest, shoulders, abdomen, quadriceps, and hip flexors. It engages the glutes, hamstrings, and back muscles—not to mention it's a great full-body energizer! It's a great pose to do if you sit at a desk or feel tight in your upper body.

The Practice Lie on your belly with your arms alongside you, palms turned in toward your body. Squeeze your thighs together, and bend your knees. Reach back with your hands to grab hold of the outsides of your feet or ankles. On an inhale, press your feet back against your hands and draw your shoulder blades together to lift your thighs and chest away from the floor. Broaden your collarbones, lift your sternum, and lengthen up through the crown of your head, keeping your neck long.

Stay three to five breaths, then lower down and release your legs with control.

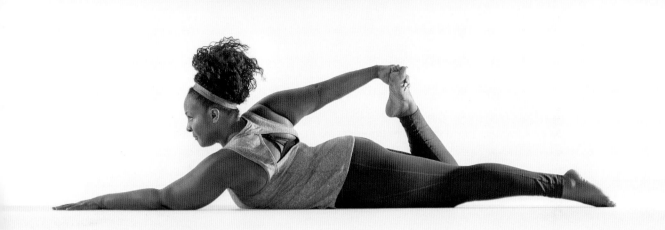

VARIATION 1: HALF BOW POSE (ARDHA DHANURASANA)

Half bow is an excellent option if you are unable to reach back and grab hold of both feet at the same time, or if doing so is uncomfortable. Begin lying face down with both arms relaxed at your sides and palms turned in toward your body. Then, prop yourself up on your left forearm to lift your torso. Bend your right knee to bring your right heel toward your bottom. Reach back with your right hand and grab hold of your right foot or ankle. Press your pelvis into the floor and, on an inhale, press your right foot or ankle against your hand and lift your chest away from the floor. Stay three to five breaths, broadening through your chest and kicking back through your right foot (keep your left foot on the floor). Release on an exhale, then change sides.

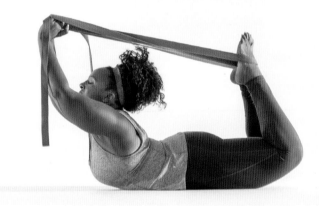

VARIATION 2: WITH STRAPS

To prepare, start seated on the floor with two straps in hand. Make a small loop (just large enough to loop around a foot) with each strap. Place each foot into a strap and tighten the loop around the arch of the foot. Then, lie on your belly to set up for bow, bending your knees and bringing the tail of each strap over its corresponding shoulder. Holding one strap in each hand, start to adjust the length of the straps by walking your hands down them until they feel taut. Once the straps are tight enough, begin to pull up on them, lifting your feet to the sky and broadening your chest. Press down through your pelvis as you continue to pull upward on the straps. Lift your gaze forward and extend out through the top of your head. Stay three to five breaths, then walk your hands forward on the straps, releasing their tension so you can lower your legs, chest, and arms to the floor with control.

BRIDGE POSE (Setu Bandha)

Setu bandha is also referred to as *setu bandha sarvanghasana*. *Sarvanghasana* means "all-limb pose," and is the Sanskrit name for shoulderstand (a yoga pose not featured in this book). While bridge does somewhat resemble shoulderstand (and is often the pose one comes into first when entering shoulderstand), it's typically thought of as a "prep" for *urdhva dhanurasana*, or wheel pose (see page 147). You can work with it as a chest and shoulder stretch, a feel-good restorative pose, or something in between.

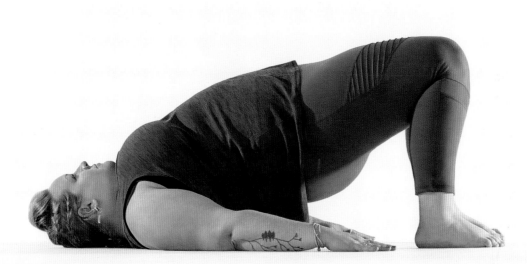

Benefits Bridge pose is what yoga teachers often refer to as a "heart opener." That means it stretches the chest and shoulders. Bridge is also a good stretch for the thighs and hip flexors.

The Practice Begin by lying on your back with your knees bent and feet flat on the floor, heels beneath your knees. Have your feet parallel if possible, and aim to keep your knees in line with the centers of your feet. Bring your arms alongside you. Draw your shoulder blades toward each other to broaden the front of your chest and shoulders. Make sure there's space between the back of your neck and the floor. Inhale here, and on an exhale, lift your hips toward the ceiling.

If available, clasp your hands beneath you and walk your shoulder blades closer together. If the back of your neck flattens toward your mat, lift your chin slightly to maintain space between your neck and the mat. Stay three to five breaths, then release your hands if they're clasped and lower your pelvis to the floor.

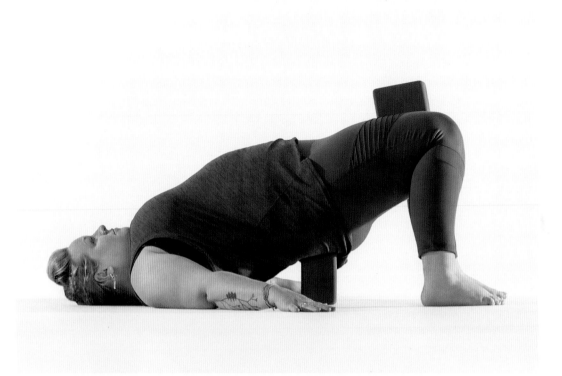

VARIATION: BLOCK-SUPPORTED BRIDGE

To enhance the restorative properties of bridge, place a block underneath your pelvis. The "sweet spot" varies from person to person—some people like the block closer to their tailbone, others prefer it more under the sacrum, which sits above the tailbone—but make sure it's under your pelvis and not your lower back. The block can be on its lowest, medium, or highest setting. You may find that you can and want to stay here longer than an unsupported bridge pose.

TIP You can squeeze a block between your thighs and/or feet to keep your knees and feet from splaying out. If clasping your hands is difficult, or if you want to try something new, try grabbing hold of the outer edges of your mat and then walking your shoulder blades closer together.

UPWARD BOW POSE (Urdhva Dhanurasana)

Also known as "wheel pose," upward bow is one of the deeper backbending postures found in typical yoga class. It requires, among other things, a lot of arm strength and power, strength from the back of the body, and flexibility in the front of the body. Wheel doesn't always feel accessible and takes a lot of time and effort to learn. Here we offer a few of our favorite variations for you.

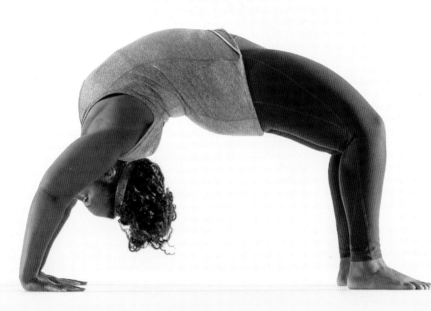

Benefits Wheel stretches the whole front of the body including the chest, shoulders, abs, hip flexors, and quads while engaging the muscles of the back of the body such as the glutes, hamstrings, and spinal muscles. For many, the pose can have an overall energizing effect, enlivening your mind and body!

The Practice Begin by lying on your back with your knees bent and feet flat on the floor. Arrange your feet so your heels are under your knees and your feet are more or less parallel to each other. Bend your elbows and bring the palms of your hands to the floor, next to your ears with your fingertips pointing toward your feet. Hug your elbows in toward each other to keep them from splaying.

On an inhale, press down into your hands and feet as you lift your shoulders and hips away from the floor. Instead of pressing all the way up right away, bring the crown of your head to the mat. Pause here for a moment. Do you need to widen your hands a little? Make any adjustments you need to feel as strong and stable as possible here. Keep hugging your elbows in and plug your arm bones into the shoulder sockets.

On your next inhale, press down through your legs and feet as you straighten your arms and lift your head off the floor. Relax your neck. Adjust your feet as needed to keep them more or less parallel with your knees and toes pointing in the same direction. If you feel comfortable here, you can lift onto the balls of your feet and walk your feet closer to your hands. Then, lower your heels with control and without letting your feet turn out. Root down through your feet and press your chest back through your arms, toward the wall behind you.

Hold for three to five breaths. To come out, walk your feet forward if you walked them back, then tuck your chin and lower the back of your shoulders and your upper back onto the mat first as you come down.

TIP If you feel restricted by tight quads, try keeping your heels lifted in wheel.

VARIATION 1: WHEEL AT THE WALL

Place a rolled blanket or small bolster against the baseboard of the wall. Lie on your back with your head pointing toward the wall in front of the blanket or bolster (do not place your head on the blanket or bolster), knees bent, and feet flat on the floor, as in the previous variation. Place your hands on the blanket or bolster with your fingertips pointing toward your feet. Resist your elbows in toward each other to keep them from splaying. Press down through your feet and push your prop against the wall as you lift your hips and shoulders off the floor. Come onto the crown of your head first so that you can check in and make any adjustments needed in your hands and feet. Then, on an inhale, press into your feet and hands as you straighten your arms and lift your head away from the floor.

As you hold wheel, continue to press your feet into the floor, your hands into your prop, and your prop against the wall. Keep your head and neck relaxed, and press your chest back toward the wall. Stay three to five breaths, then tuck your chin to come down, lowering the backs of your shoulders and your upper back first.

TIP You can also try this variation with blocks under your hands. If your legs are on the shorter side and/or your quads and hip flexors feel tight, you might try propping up your feet instead of your hands.

VARIATION 2: WHEEL STANDING AT THE WALL

Stand with your back to the wall, about twelve inches away from it. Separate your feet hip-width apart, place your hands on your hips, and root down through your feet. Resist your feet apart from each other to activate your legs. Lengthen up through the crown of your head and draw your shoulder blades together onto your back. Then, reach your arms up and back, bringing your hands to touch the wall behind you. Walk your hands down the wall as you walk your feet away from the wall until your chest is curling up toward the sky. Take your gaze upward. Stay three to five breaths. Come out of the pose on an inhale: walk your feet back toward the wall if you walked them forward quite a bit, push the wall away from you, and lead with your chest as you rise back up to standing upright.

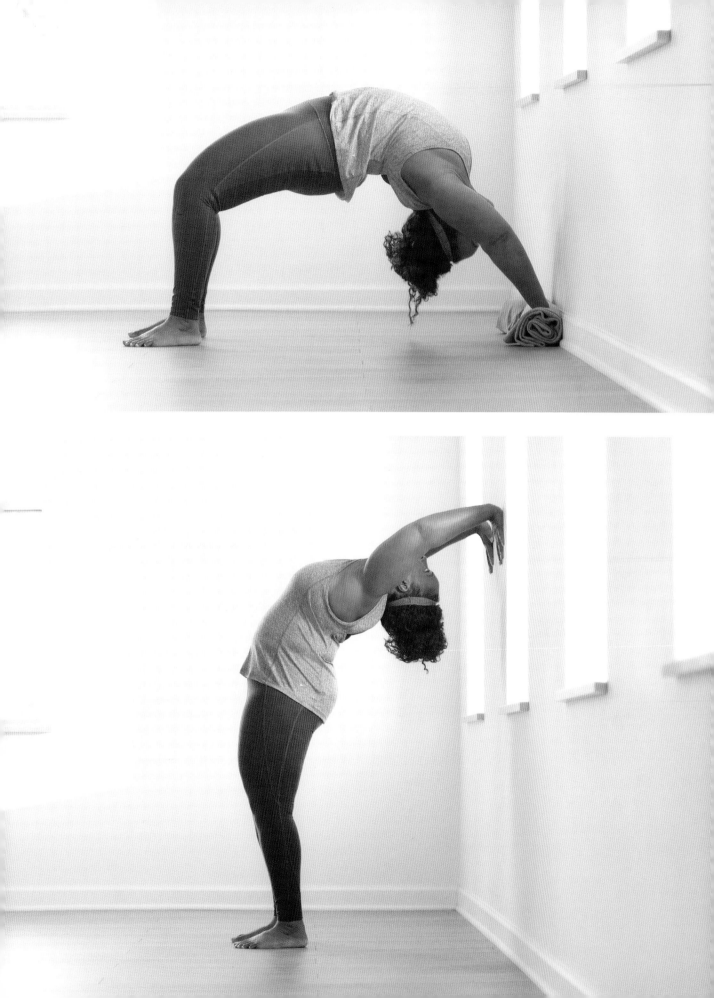

VARIATION 3: STONEHENGE SETUP

For this variation, you'll use blocks and a firm bolster to build a platform to support you. You can also use this setup to get into a straight-arm, unsupported wheel pose: it gives you a little extra "lift" from the get-go and can make the "traditional" version of wheel more accessible.

Place a block on its lowest setting underneath each end of your bolster. Sit on the edge of the bolster with your feet flat on the floor, and use your hands to help you lie all the way back on the bolster and gently lower your head toward the floor. Plant your hands by your ears with your fingertips pointing toward your shoulders.

Press into your hands and draw your shoulder blades onto your back. Try pressing up and lifting yourself a few centimeters from the bolster. Lower down and try again.

If you want to come up into a straight-armed urdhva dhanurasana, on an inhale, lift your hips and straighten your arms to press all the way up. Root down through your legs and feet and press your chest back through your arms, keeping your head and neck relaxed. Stay a few breaths if you're comfortable here, then tuck your chin and bend your elbows to lower back onto the bolster.

You can either roll onto one side and off the bolster to come out or press your hands into the floor and rise up to a seated position.

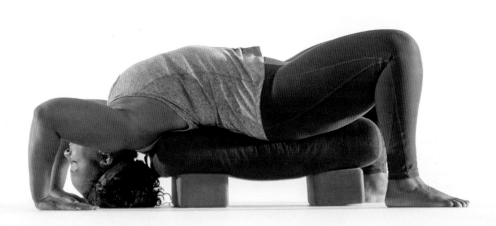

WILD THING (Chamatkarasana)

Also known as "flip dog," wild thing has become a staple in vinyasa classes in recent years. Even though it goes by a Sanskrit moniker that translates as "astonishment, surprise spectacle," or, our favorite, "festive turbulence," this asana is relatively new—according to most accounts, first showing up in the yogaverse somewhere in the 1990s. While the idea of flipping into it from downward-facing dog can be scary, it's a favorite of many yoga practitioners, perhaps due in part to its playful, expressive nature.

Benefits Like all backbends, wild thing offers a chest and shoulder stretch. It also provides a nice stretch for your hip flexors, and, depending on how you enter into it, can be a great way to work with core strength and shoulder stability.

The Practice Before we explore the common "flip dog" entrance, let's look at coming into wild thing from side plank, an entrance that is often more accessible and less taxing on the shoulders.

Begin in side plank (see page 176) on your left side (left hand down). Make sure your left wrist crease is parallel with the short edge of your mat, and that the eye of your left elbow is pointing toward the space between your index finger and thumb. From there, bend your right knee and *lightly* rest the ball of your right foot on the floor behind your left leg. Then, reach your right arm up alongside your ear, spinning the pinky side of the hand toward the floor. If you like, you can stay in this "side bendy" version of wild thing, gazing down toward your left hand, straight ahead, or up toward your right hand.

Or, you can spin your chest up toward the ceiling, turning the pose into more of a backbend, and perhaps planting your left foot on the floor. Expand through your chest, release your head back if it feels good, and make your expression of the pose as wild as you want! For added challenge, experiment with hovering your right toes away from the floor. To exit, return to side plank, or plant your right hand on the ground to come into downward dog. Then switch sides.

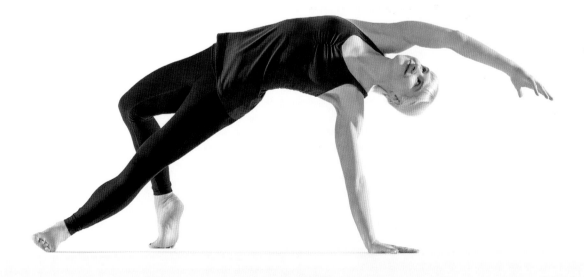

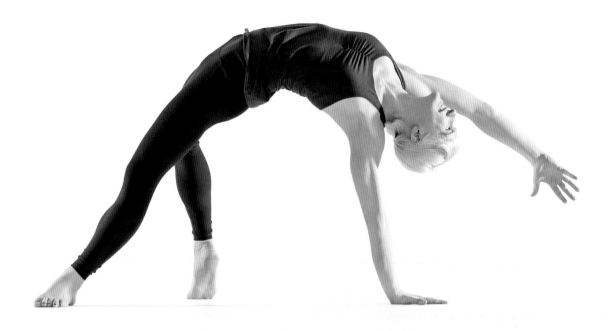

Flip Dog Entrance

To come into wild thing from downward dog, lift your right leg to the sky (this position is often referred to as "three-legged dog") and bend your right knee, stacking your right hip over your left. This "open hip" position is sometimes referred to as "scorpion dog." Notice how your right hand gets light on your mat. If you were to stay in scorpion dog, you might want to press more weight into your right hand so that your shoulders remain level and you can really focus on "opening" your right hip. However, if you're going to flip into wild thing, instead of pressing into your right hand, let it lift away from the floor as you bring the ball of your right foot to (*lightly*) rest on the floor behind your left leg and spin your chest up toward the sky. Hello, wild thing!

To exit, plant your right hand and return to downward dog. Then switch sides.

VARIATION 1: KNEELING WILD THING

This variation allows you to press right into your backbend, which can be easier on your shoulders. It's also lower to the ground, which can make wild thing feel more approachable.

To try it, begin in a "Z-sit" with your left shin forward and your right leg back, bringing the sole of your left foot to rest on or near your right inner thigh, just below the knee. From here, plant your left hand a foot or so behind your left hip with your fingers pointing back (far enough away so that when you lift up, your left shoulder will be directly over or a little bit behind your left wrist). On an inhale, lift your hips away from the floor and stretch your right arm overhead, opening your chest toward the sky. Gaze up or wherever feels most comfortable. Enjoy a few breaths here, then lower your hips down and switch sides.

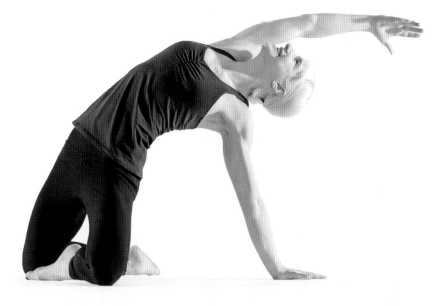

VARIATION 2: STARGAZER

Like the previous variation, you'll press up into this one from the ground. Stargazer can be particularly nice to come into after janu sirsasana (see page 134).

Begin seated with your right leg straight and your left leg bent with the ball of your left foot resting on or near your right inner thigh. From here, plant your left hand on the floor, about a foot or so behind your left hip, with your fingers pointing away from you, and press up, lifting your hips off the floor, opening your chest toward the sky, and sweeping your right arm up overhead. The sole of your right foot can come to the floor.

When you're ready, lower your hips and switch sides.

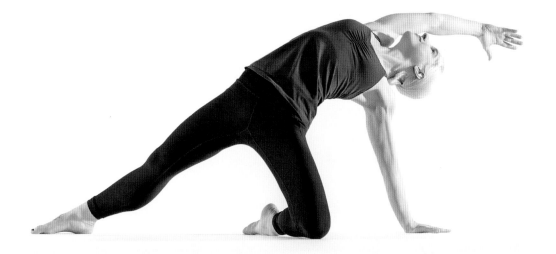

MERMAID POSE (Naginyasana)

Mermaid is a close cousin to, and sometimes considered a variation of, pigeon pose (see page 111). For many people, mermaid is more accessible than other backbending forms of pigeon, which often require you to reach your arms up overhead to catch hold of your back foot—a feat that requires more shoulder and spine mobility than the average person possesses.

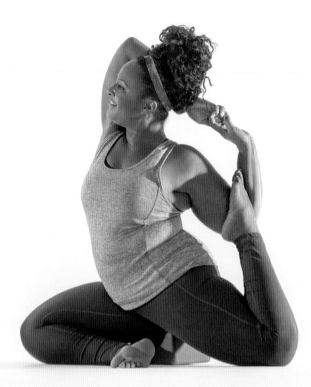

Benefits Mermaid is a great stretch for your hips, groin, quadriceps, hip flexors, chest, shoulders, biceps, and triceps. Like King Arthur pose (see page 107), because your back knee is bent you get a stretch for *all* of your quadriceps—including the vastus lateralis, vastus medialis, and vastus intermedius muscles, which cross the knee joint and often get left out in pigeon variations where the back leg is straight.

The Practice Begin in pigeon with your right leg forward and your right shin as close to parallel with the top of the mat as is comfortable. Because it can be challenging to find balance when coming into the pose, we like to place a block underneath the right hip for support.

Press your fingertips into the floor and lift your torso away from your thigh, lengthening the front of your body.

From here, bend your left knee, bringing your heel toward your bottom. Reach your left hand back and clasp the inner edge of your left foot. Then, see if you can bring your left foot inside of your left forearm. Draw your foot closer toward your body until your foot comes to the crease of your left elbow. Press your foot into your arm and bring it closer to you.

With your spine long, reach your right arm overhead and back behind you. Bend your right elbow and reach your right forearm behind your head and clasping your left hand with your right. Square your torso toward the front of your mat. Stay for three to five breaths, then release with control and change sides.

VARIATION 1: THIGH STRETCH WITH NO BIND

If it feels better in your body, you can skip the elbow bind but still cash in on the thigh-stretchy goodness of mermaid.

You may wish to place a block under your right hip to support your balance. Keep your torso upright, pressing your fingertips into the floor on either side of you to begin. Then, bend your left knee to draw your left heel in toward your seat and catch hold of the big-toe side of your foot (holding the big-toe side will make it easier to keep your left shoulder rolling back instead of forward, allowing you to experience

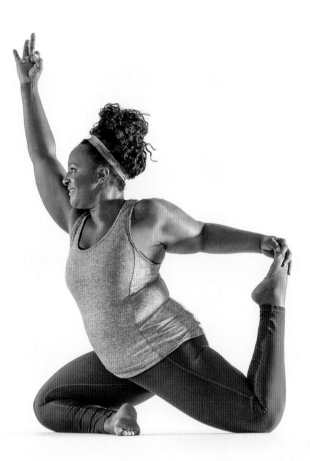

more chest opening). Turn your chest to face forward and bend your left elbow to draw your heel closer to your seat. Keep your right fingertips on the floor or, for added balance challenge, reach your right arm up. Stay three to five breaths.

To come out, return your right fingertips to the floor if your arm was lifted and release your back foot with control. Switch sides.

VARIATION 2: THIGH STRETCH WITH A TWIST

Some people find that adding a twist enhances the quad and hip-flexor stretch in the back leg. Set up as in the previous variation, bending your back (left) knee to draw your heel in toward your seat, but instead of catching hold of the big-toe side of the foot with your left hand, catch hold of the pinky-toe side of your foot with your right hand. It might feel good to bring your left forearm to the floor, as Dianne is demonstrating, or to a prop in front of you here, or you can remain more upright. Spin your chest open to the right as you draw your left heel in toward your seat. Gaze in whatever direction feels best for your neck. Stay three to five breaths.

To exit, release your back foot with control, and unwind to face forward in pigeon where you began. Then switch sides.

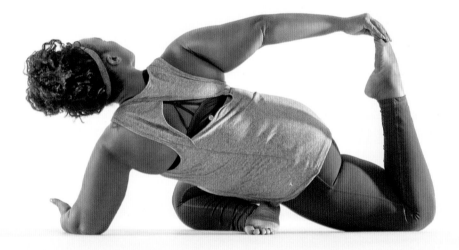

11

Inversions

DOLPHIN POSE (Ardha Pincha Mayurasana)
+ FOREARM BALANCE (Pincha Mayurasana)

Dolphin is a variation of downward dog that is done on the forearms. It's an excellent alternative to down-dog if you have sore wrists, but dolphin can be difficult if you have sore or tight shoulders. Dolphin pose—*ardha pincha mayurasana*—is also a preparation for *pincha mayurasana*, forearm balance, which we delve into here as well!

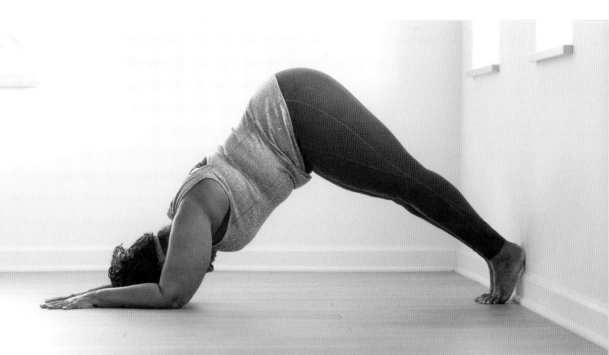

Benefits Dolphin strengthens the upper back and shoulders and stretches the glutes, hamstrings, and calves.

The Practice Begin on hands and knees, then lower your elbows to the floor directly beneath your shoulders. Keep your forearms parallel to each other and to the edges of your mat. Press weight down through your forearms. Tuck your toes and lift your knees from the floor, coming to an inverted V shape. Keep your head in line with your spine. Lengthen through your spine as much as possible (bending your knees can help). Stay three to five breaths, then lower your knees to release.

TIP If your elbows splay out, try bringing your hands together in a prayer position, clasping your hands as you would for headstand (see page 161) or holding a block between your hands.

You can also do dolphin with your heels pressing into a wall (as Dianne is demonstrating in the photo) for an added sense of support and feedback. Set up on forearms and knees with your toes tucked and the balls of your feet making contact with the baseboard, and then lift your knees and press back into dolphin from there.

If you are working toward forearm balance, you can start to walk your legs up the wall. (You may need to adjust your positioning a bit, perhaps lowering down and coming a little closer to the wall, so that your shoulders are stacked right over your elbows when you come up.) Walk your legs up the wall until your legs are parallel to the floor. This pose is very similar to L handstand at the wall (see page 165), except your forearms are on the ground.

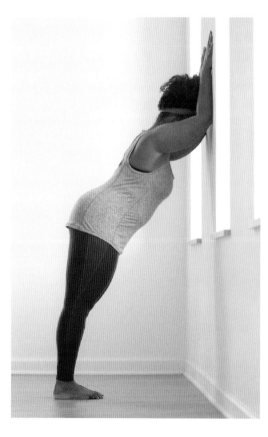

VARIATION 1: WITH FOREARMS ON THE WALL

Begin standing, facing the wall. Lean forward and place your forearms on the wall with your elbows at or slightly above shoulder height. Press your forearms into the wall and walk your feet back a few inches. Aim to find as much length through your spine as possible and keep your head in line with your spine. Stay three to five breaths, then walk back in toward the wall and release your arms to come out.

You can experiment with moving your feet farther away from the wall if you like, bringing your torso more parallel with the floor.

VARIATION 2: WITH FOREARMS ON A CHAIR SEAT

Begin by standing in front of the seat. Your feet can be hip-width apart, or closer, or wider, depending on what feels best. Fold forward from your hip creases and bring your elbows and forearms onto the seat. For support, wrap

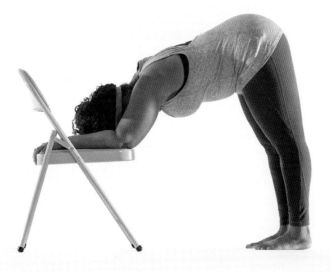

your fingers around the back of the seat of the chair. Walk your feet back away from the seat of the chair, keeping your spine long as you find your dolphin pose. Stay three to five breaths, then walk your feet forward to come out.

TIP Walk your feet farther from the chair to create a more significant stretch in the legs and recruit more engagement in the shoulders. Move the feet closer to the chair to create more stability in the pose.

VARIATION 3: KNEELING DOLPHIN WITH A CHAIR

This is another excellent way to make dolphin more accessible. Begin by kneeling facing the seat. You can place a blanket on it and/or beneath your knees to make the pose more comfortable. Place the back of your upper arms, just above your elbows, on the seat. Now, walk your knees back so they're just below your hips. Rest your forehead on the chair seat. Bring your hands together in prayer behind your head. Draw your shoulder blades together. Find as much length through your spine as you can here and stay for several relaxed breaths. Then bring your hands to the chair seat to come out of the pose.

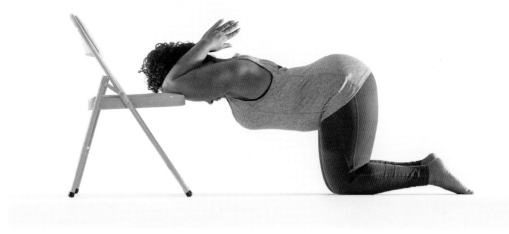

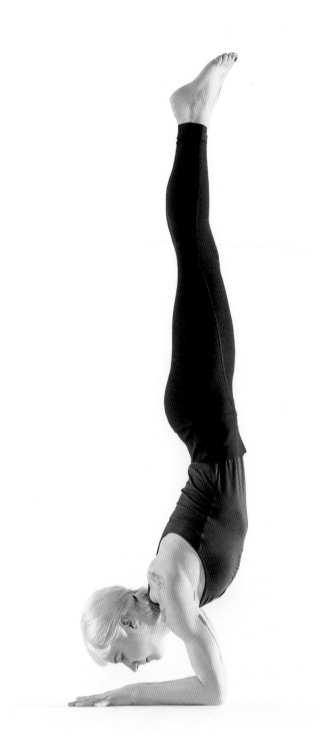

VARIATION 4: FOREARM BALANCE, PEACOCK TAIL-FEATHER POSE (PINCHA MAYURASANA)

Forearm balance can seem less intimidating if you think of it as a dolphin variation—a dolphin going for a dive perhaps!

To set up, begin in dolphin. If you're new to forearm stand or worried about flipping over, practice in front of a wall. Set up your arms as in dolphin (described above) using any of the arm variations if preferred to help keep your elbows under your shoulders.

Keeping your shoulders stacked over your elbows, walk your feet as close to your elbows as you can. Resist your outer forearms in toward each other and press your forearms, wrists, and hands into the floor. Gaze forward toward your hands, or wherever is comfortable. On an inhale, lift one leg into the air (don't worry about keeping your hips square; it's okay if they open up a little) and rise onto the ball of your bottom foot. On an exhale, bend your bottom knee and try to hop up, bringing your bottom foot to meet your top foot. It may take you a few hops to get up, or you might not come up at all and simply stick with the hopping for now.

If you arrive in *pincha mayurasana*, continue to hug your forearms in and push the floor away.

Reach up through your inner heels if your feet are flexed or "flointed" (or feel free to point your toes if that feels best). Keep your neck long and gaze toward your thumbs or anywhere that feels comfortable and stable. If you're practicing at a wall, experiment with lifting one—or both—feet away from it.

Lower one leg at a time to come down, and then try hopping up with the opposite leg lifted.

HEADSTAND (Sirsasana)

Headstand is often referred to as the "king" of poses. This gives the impression that it's pretty important, right? The problem is, headstand can also be scary for new and even experienced students. Not to mention that for some of us, bearing weight on our heads is contraindicated. The solution? Unpacking the pose and figuring out how to make it work for *you*. Here, we offer some tips and instructions for a traditional form of headstand and also some variations that offer all of the same benefits but don't involve bearing any weight on your head.

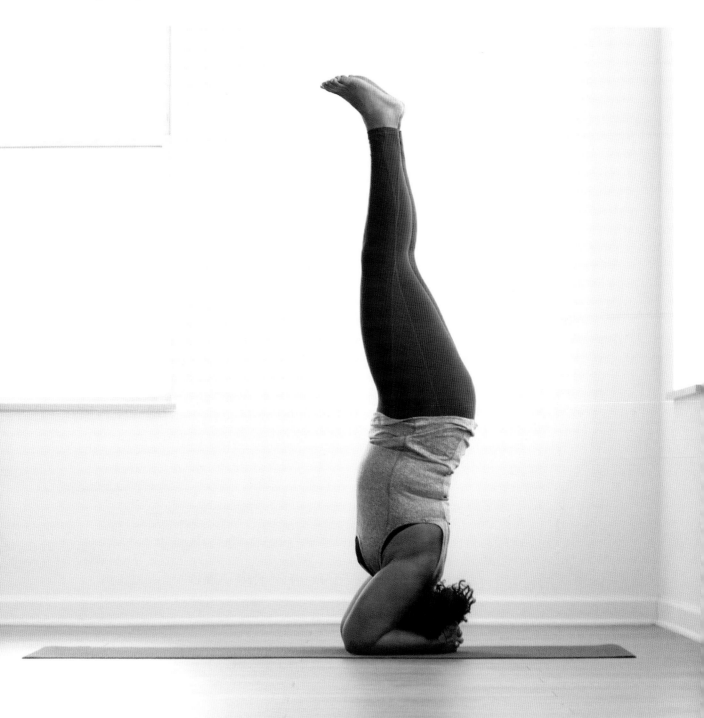

Benefits One of the biggest advantages of inversions like headstand is that they can build confidence. Headstand can be daunting at first. The fear of falling is real, but once you get past that fear, this pose can lift your spirits and change your perspective.

The Practice Begin on hands and knees, facing a wall for an added sense of security if you like. Lower your forearms to the floor with your elbows just below your shoulders. Interlace your fingers, tucking your bottom pinky finger into your palms so that you can press the outer edges of your hands, your forearms, and your wrists firmly into the floor. Place the crown of your head on the floor behind your clasped hands.

Pressing firmly into the floor, lift your knees and walk your feet toward your elbows. When your feet are close enough to allow you to, on an exhale draw both knees into your chest. Pause here and find your balance. Engage your abdominals and hug your thighs toward each other. When you feel balanced, straighten your legs toward the sky. Firm your outer arms toward each other and push the floor away from you. Continue to hug your legs together and press out through your heels.

Stay for five to ten breaths or as long as you feel stable. To come down, bend your knees into your chest, then lower your toes to the floor, lower your knees down, and untuck your toes and sit back on your heels to rest in child's pose.

VARIATION 1: HEADLESS HEADSTAND WITH STONEHENGE SETUP

This variation doesn't require you to put any weight on your head, making it a great headstand alternative and also a great prep for, or variation of, forearm balance (see page 157). The block setup gives you something to press into, helping you to find your balance with your feet away from the wall.

You'll need three blocks and some open wall space. Scoot one of the short edges of your mat against the wall and set up one block, on its tallest setting, an inch or so away from the wall with the longer, narrower side of the block facing the wall. Stack the other two blocks on top of the first block, on their flattest vertical settings. The top two blocks should be touching the wall.

Once your blocks are set up, come onto forearms and knees and interlace your hands around the bottom block (adjusting its position a bit if necessary, though be sure the top blocks remain in contact with the wall). Stack your shoulders over your elbows. Resist your forearms in toward each other and push them into the floor. Maintain those actions as you tuck your toes and press up to dolphin pose. Keeping your shoulders stacked over your elbows and your head away from the floor, walk your feet toward the wall until your upper back lightly touches the blocks.

From here, lift one leg, bend your standing leg knee, and see if you can hop up into a forearm balance, bringing your heels to touch the wall to begin. If the back of your head is touching the bottom block, you can gently press into it. This, in addition to gently pressing your upper back into the top two blocks, can help you find more balance and core activation in the pose. If you feel stable, you can experiment with moving one, maybe both, heels off the wall.

If you regularly practice headstand and your proportions allow, you could allow your crown to *lightly* rest on the floor. Otherwise, keep your head hovering away from the floor. Stay for three to five breaths, then lower one leg at a time to come down.

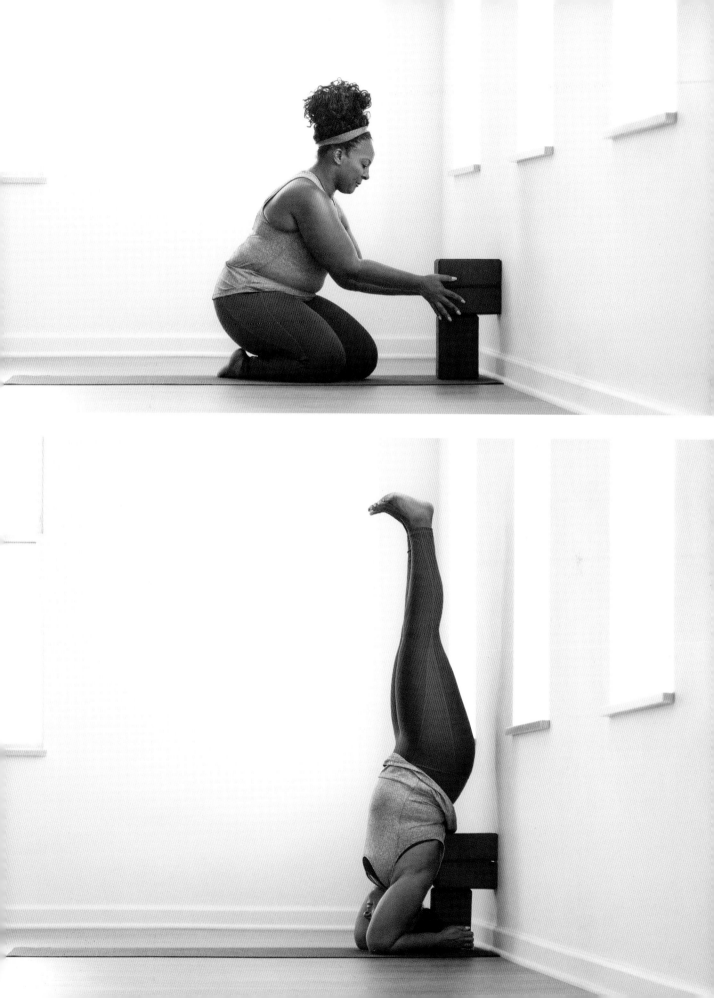

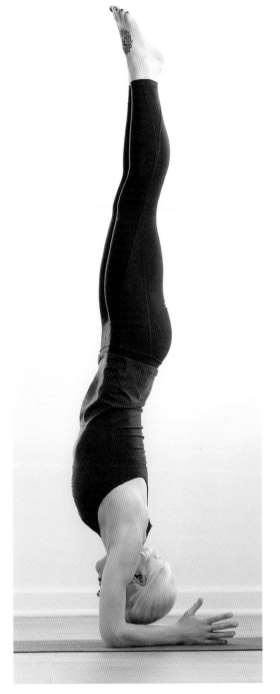

VARIATION 2: HEADLESS HEADSTAND AWAY FROM THE WALL

Like the "Stonehenge" variation, this version doesn't put any weight on your head, but it removes the support of the blocks, requiring you to rely more on your own balance and recruit more core and shoulder strength.

From all fours, lower to your forearms, stacking your shoulders above your elbows. Either clasp your hands or bring them into prayer position (as with sirsasana, if you clasp your hands, tuck in your bottom pinky). Then, tuck your toes and lift your hips to come into dolphin. Keeping your shoulders stacked over your elbows, walk your feet toward your elbows, as close as you can without collapsing into your shoulders. Gaze back toward your legs. Resist your forearms toward each other while simultaneously pressing them into the floor. Keep your head lifted away from the floor. From here, lift a leg, bend the knee of your standing leg, and hop up into a forearm balance. Keep hugging your forearms toward each other and pushing the floor away from you. Instead of gazing toward your hands, tuck your chin slightly so your crown is facing (but hovering above!) the floor. Stay three to five breaths, then lower one leg at a time to come down.

HANDSTAND (Adho Mukha Vriksasana)

Adho mukha vriksasana (upward-facing tree pose, more commonly known as handstand) is rife with opportunities to explore but figuring out just where to begin, or where to go next, can be a challenge. There are lots of ways to approach handstand, and here we'll explore ways to "walk" up into it and hop up into it, and we'll look at a few drills for "floating" into handstand too (and explain exactly what yoga teachers mean when they talk about "floating").

Benefits Handstand both requires and builds wrist, arm, shoulder, and core strength.

The Practice

Walking into Handstand

Walking up the wall into a handstand requires a good amount of upper body strength, but it can be a great starting place for a handstand practice because you have a lot of control over the transition (unlike hopping or jumping into a handstand where you might be more likely to "overshoot" and flip over into wheel pose!).

VARIATION 1: L POSE AT THE WALL

Begin by sitting facing a wall with your legs extended in front of you and your feet on the baseboard. Place your hands beside your hips. Noting where your hands are, flip over onto hands and knees and place your hands right where they were before. Make sure your outer shoulders are aligned with the centers of your wrists, your fingers are spread comfortably and evenly apart, and that the creases of your wrists are parallel with the short edge of your mat.

Tuck your toes, lift your knees, and walk your feet back to the baseboard. This will feel like a short downward dog with your heels pressed into the wall. Pressing the floor away from you, step one foot up the wall at hip height and then the other. Press your feet into the wall and lift your inner thighs toward the ceiling. Take your gaze toward the baseboard. Aim to stay for three breaths, then walk your feet down the wall to come out.

Hopping into Handstand

If you're newer to handstand or concerned about flipping over, we recommend practicing at the wall. Bring the short edge of your mat to the wall and set up with your fingertips a few inches away from it. The more comfortable you get with your balance, the farther you can set up away from the wall.

VARIATION 2: ONE KNEE BENT

Set up on all fours with your shoulders over your wrists, knees under your hips, and toes tucked. Press your hips up and back to come into a short downward dog. Step one foot forward so there's about a foot of space between your foot and your hands.

Lift your back leg up and rise up onto the ball of your front foot, shifting your shoulders forward so that they're stacked directly over, or slightly forward of, your wrists. (Feel free to adjust the position of your bottom foot as needed.) Gaze toward your thumbs.

This is your starting position for handstand hops. Don't worry about keeping your hips square here; it's okay to let your lifted leg turn out.

Before you start hopping, try this prep: Inhale, and on an exhale, bend your standing-leg knee and tap your lifted-leg toes down to the floor. Inhale, straighten your standing leg, and lift your back leg back up. Repeat a few more times:

Exhale, bend and tap.
Inhale, lift.

When you're ready, you can add in the hop:

Inhale, lift your back leg.
Exhale, bend and tap.

Then, briefly suspend the exhale and hop up, bending your hopping-leg knee in toward your chest and keeping your back leg straight. Repeat a few more times:

Inhale, lift.
Exhale, tap.
Pause on the exhale and hop up.

If hopping up on the suspension (pause) after the exhale feels awkward, you can instead hop up on the exhale:

Inhale, lift.
Exhale, tap and hop.

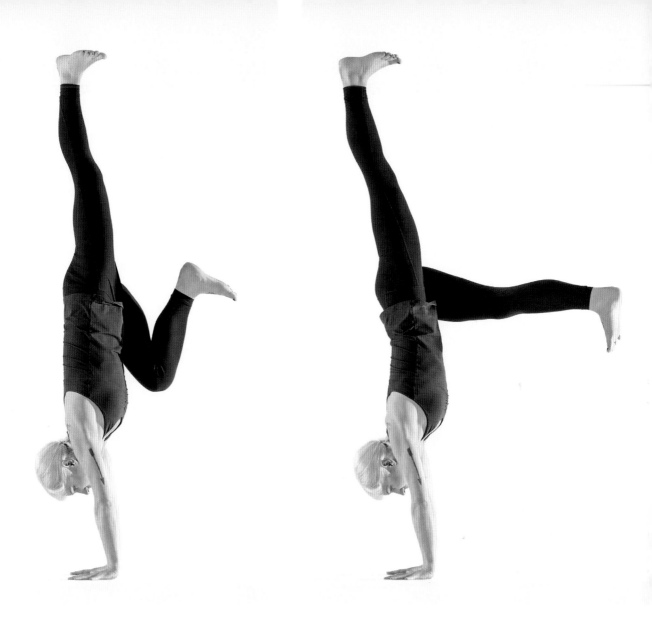

You can stick with the hops, or try to catch some hang time in your handstand, keeping one knee bent or stretching that leg straight up to meet your other leg. Lower one leg at a time to come down.

VARIATION 3: BOTH LEGS STRAIGHT

As in the previous variation, begin on all fours, press up into a short downward dog, and step one foot forward so there's about a foot of space between your foot and hands.

Lift your back leg and rise onto the ball of your front foot, shifting your shoulders over, or slightly forward of your wrists.

For this variation, you'll keep your hips relatively square to the floor and instead of tapping your back toes down, you'll keep your back leg lifted.

Inhale, and as you exhale, bend your bottom-leg knee slightly and then hop up, leading with your hips to come into a handstand with your legs making an L shape.

Here too, stick with the hopping, or maybe catch some hang time and hold your handstand. If you do, you can keep the L shape or bring your bottom leg to meet your top leg in a straight up-and-down handstand.

Floating up to Handstand

Have you ever heard a yoga teacher say to "hop, jump, or float into handstand"? Or maybe, "float forward to the top of your mat from down-dog"? What does that mean? Is a float really any different than a jump?

While different teachers and schools of yoga all have their own terminology, in general, the difference between a float and a jump is that when you "float" you have a little bit of "hover" or "hang time."

If you're "floating" from downward dog to a forward bend, for example, you jump up off two feet and shift lots of weight into your fingertips so your feet can hover away from the floor (maybe tapping your wrists) before softly landing on the ground behind your wrists.

If you're floating into a handstand, instead of lowering your feet to the ground, from that hover, you raise them up into the air. In this way, a "float" into handstand is closely related to a handstand press: where you place your hands on the floor, rise up onto your toes, shift your weight into your fingertips, and push the floor away with your hands as you lift your feet from the floor to rise into handstand without momentum.

Whether you're working on floating or pressing into handstand, or you just want to try something new, these two "float" drills can be a great addition to your practice.

For prep 1, one foot will always remain on the wall. You'll want to be pretty comfortable practicing L handstand at the wall before trying it. For prep 2, both feet will come off the wall, so you'll want to be very comfortable with a middle-of-the-room handstand before trying it.

Prep 1: Toe Taps

Begin by coming into L handstand, as described above in variation 1. Once you're there, gaze forward, between your thumbs. Exhale, bend your right knee (the ball of your right foot will stay on the wall and your right heel will lift away) and, keeping your left leg straight, bring your left toes to tap the back of your left wrist. Inhale, push the floor away with your hands as you straighten your right leg (your right heel will come back to the wall), and lift your left leg back up to hip height without touching the wall with your left foot.

Try three to five reps on this side, take a break, and then switch sides.

TIP In order to tap your toes to your wrist, you *really* have to shift weight into your fingertips. In order to lift your leg back up, you *really* have to push the floor away. Both of these actions are key for floating or pressing into handstand.

Prep 2: Wall Floats

For this one, you'll begin closer to the wall than you were for L handstand. Try setting up on all fours, facing away from the wall with the heels of your hands about an arm's distance away from it. From there, walk your feet up the wall to hip height. You'll be in a squat shape with your knees bent a lot and your heels off the wall. Gaze forward, between your thumbs.

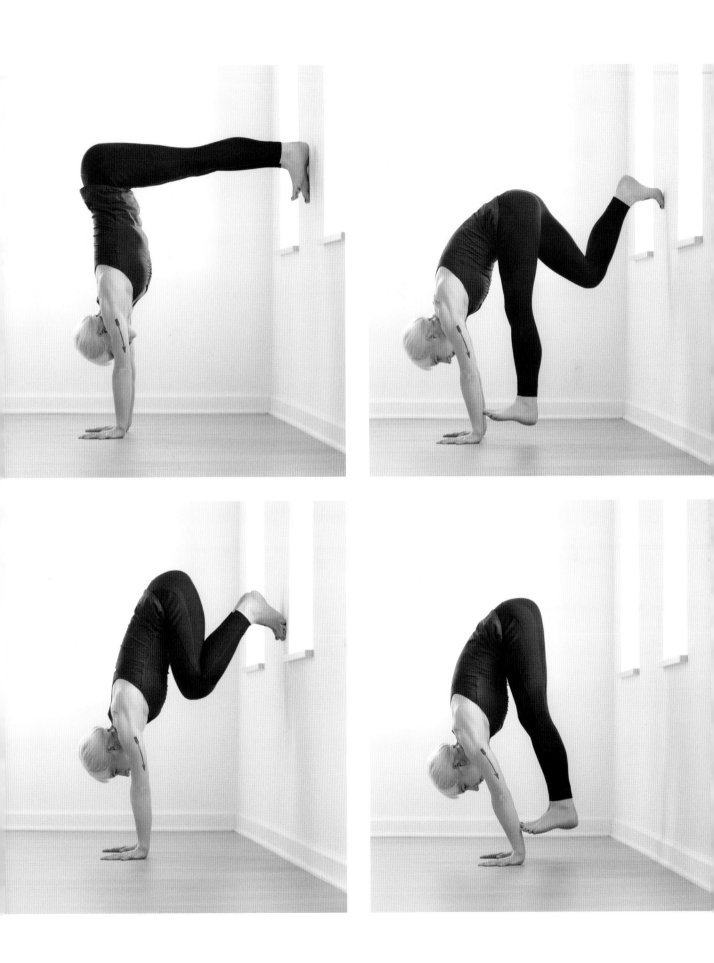

From this wall squat, shift more weight into your fingertips, so much that the heels of your hands get light on the floor, and maybe, you can float your toes off the wall and bring them to tap the backs of your wrists before bringing them back to the wall.

Try three reps to start, breathing in a way that feels natural to you (for example, you might exhale as you tap your wrists and inhale as you float your feet back to the wall).

Keep in mind: This is a *really* challenging drill. It's normal if it feels awkward, frustrating, or even impossible. Instead of floating your feet back to the wall after tapping your wrists, your feet might land on the floor behind your hands. That's totally fine! You can walk your feet back up the wall and do a few more reps just like that. Eventually, you might be able to land your feet on the wall and your floats might start to feel more "floaty." But the important thing is that you enjoy the exploration. Drills in particular are all about building strength, not about doing anything perfectly!

SCORPION POSE (Vrischikasana)

Scorpion is an arm balance combined with a backbend. It can be practiced from forearm stand (sometimes called *vrischikasana* I) or handstand (sometimes called *vrischikasana* II). Here we'll look at the forearm-stand variation, but you can apply many of these instructions to the handstand variation too.

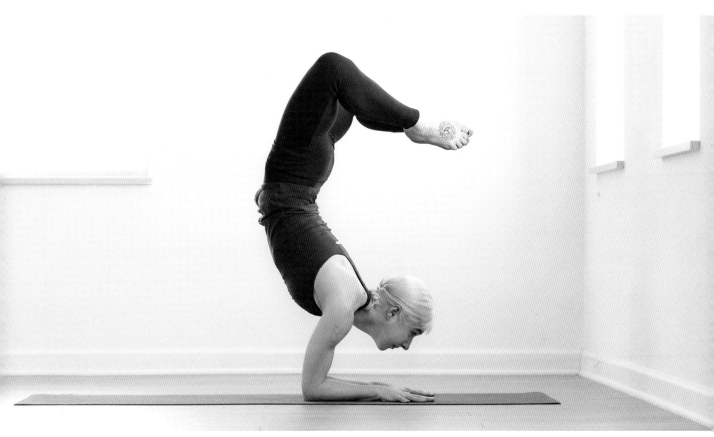

Benefits As a (fore)arm balance and backbend, this pose requires a good amount of shoulder stability/mobility, and preparing for and working with it can help to develop that. And as with any arm balance, it can also be pretty exhilarating! But as far as we're concerned, this pose's top benefit is the *fun* we have exploring it. We recommend being pretty comfortable with forearm balance (see page 157) before working with scorpion.

The Practice Come into forearm balance to start. You might find it helpful to practice near a wall. Start with your hands six inches or so away from the wall (adjusting as needed to accommodate your proportions)—close enough that your feet can touch the wall, but not so close that you can't come into the backbend. You can have forearms parallel (holding a block between your hands if you like), clasped, or in a prayer position. In forearm balance, hug your forearms in toward each other, and press them into the floor. Keep your gaze slightly toward your hands. Focus on broadening your chest and drawing it forward, as though you were drawing your chest "through" your upper arms.

Then, begin to bend your knees, allowing them to separate, but keeping your big toes touching as you draw them closer to your head. Don't worry about getting your toes to *touch* your head; that's not the point of the pose, and whether or not that's possible for you depends largely on your body proportions. As you can see in the photo here, Kat's feet are quite far away from her head despite the fact that she is in what is, for her, a very deep backbend!

If you're practicing at a wall, slide your toes down the wall as you bend and separate your knees. Perhaps your toes stay on the wall the whole time, or maybe they lift away.

When you're ready to come out, lower one leg at a time.

VARIATION 1: WITH FEET ON A CHAIR

Scorpion on a chair is still an intense backbend, but the chair makes it a little more accessible.

To begin, kneel in front of a chair facing the seat. Your exact distance from the chair will depend on your proportions and may require a little experimenting to find. Come into forearm balance (see page 157). Bring your feet to the chair seat, one then the other, with as much control as you can. Press the floor away from you with your forearms and gaze wherever feels best for your neck. Stay a few breaths if you feel stable, then lower one leg at a time to release.

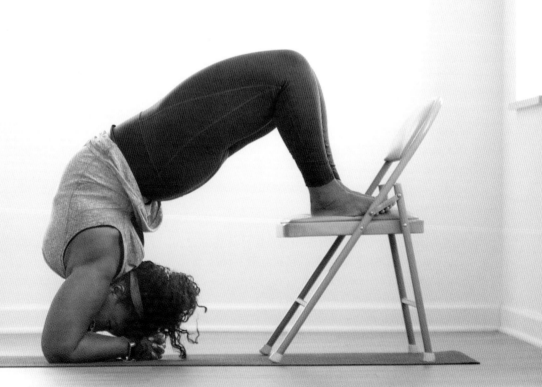

VARIATION 2: REVERSE SCORPION

This variation is sometimes called "charging scorpion" or a "hollow-back" variation because of the backbend it requires. As with previous variations, you can practice it with your forearms parallel, hands clasped, or hands in prayer.

Instead of starting in pincha mayurasana (gazing toward your hands), you're starting point is headless headstand (variation 2, page 164) with the crown of your head hovering away from the floor.

From here, bend your knees in toward your chest. Continue to push the floor away with your forearms as you draw your chest *back* through your arms and reach your hips in the opposite direction.

Stay for a few breaths, then lower one leg at a time to come down.

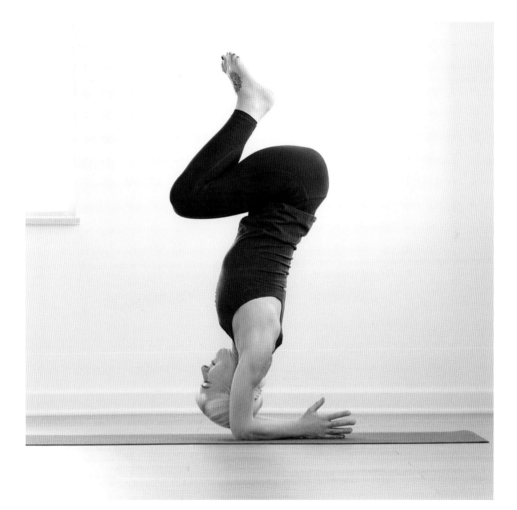

LEGS-UP-THE-WALL POSE (Viparita Karani)

Viparita karani translates to "inverted action" but is commonly referred to as legs-up-the-wall. A supported and often therapeutic option, legs-up-the-wall can be an alternative to inversions such as headstand and shoulderstand, and it can also be an excellent alternative to *savasana* during the final relaxation at the end of your practice.

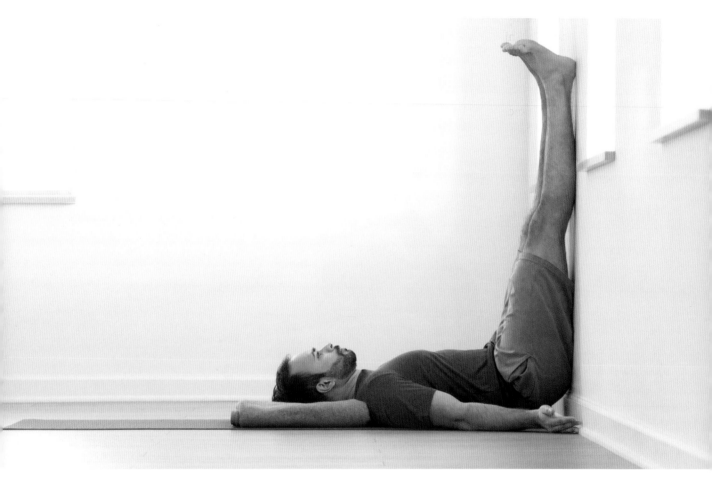

Benefits Legs-up-the-wall pose shares benefits with other inversions, such as helping you to feel rejuvenated and restored, improving your mood, calming the central nervous system, improving circulation, helping with lymph drainage, and offering sweet relief for tired legs or swollen ankles. It's a particularly great pose if you travel a lot or experience jetlag.

The Practice This pose requires a little maneuvering to get into, but we promise it's worth it. To begin, sit with your left or right side against a wall. Bring your hip as close to the baseboard as possible.

Turn your body toward the side that's against the wall to roll onto your back and bring your legs up the wall. Your legs can be slightly bent if that feels good; you can keep them neutral, or allow them to turn out slightly. The key is to find a position that feels relaxed and comfortable, where you're expending as little effort as possible.

Rest your shoulders and head on the floor, or slide a blanket under your head. If your bottom is not touching the wall shift your weight from side to side and shimmy your buttocks closer to the wall. (It's okay if there's a little space between your buttocks and the wall, but you want to get as close as you comfortably can.) Rest your arms open at your sides, palms up, or bring them to any position that feels comfortable. Close your eyes if you like, or keep your gaze soft. Remain here for as long as you like! Three to five minutes is often a good amount of time to aim for.

When you're ready to come out, bend your knees, place your feet on the wall, and roll onto one side. Enjoy a few breaths there before pressing up to seated position.

TIP Typically, an inversion is any pose in which your head is below your heart. To make viparitta karani a little more of an inversion, you can elevate your hips on a bolster or folded blanket by placing your feet flat on the wall and lifting your hips up to slide the prop underneath them.

VARIATION: LEGS-UP-THE-WALL POSE WITH A STRAP

Looping a strap around your ankles or shins can make this pose even more relaxing by allowing the legs to be supported laterally as well as from behind. Place the strap around your legs before bringing them up the wall. Make sure the strap is taut enough that your legs can relax out against it and you feel fully supported, but not so tight that it's uncomfortable.

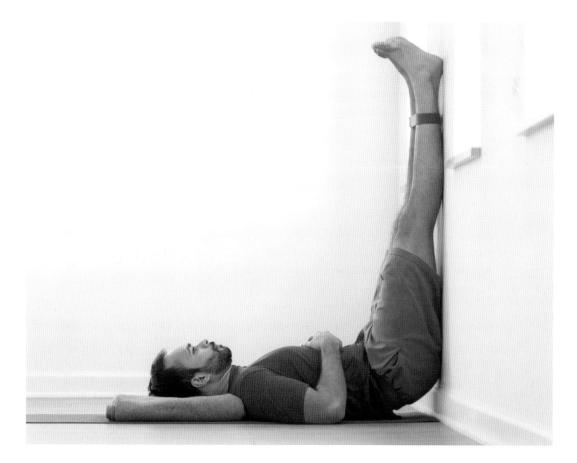

12

Arm Balances

SIDE PLANK POSE
(Vasisthasana, Pose Dedicated to Sage Vasistha)

Vasisthasana—more commonly known as side plank—is a wonderful preparation for arm balances. It takes strength, focus, and effort to balance your entire body weight on one hand and one foot.

Benefits Vasisthasana challenges your focus and your core strength. It is also an excellent pose for strengthening wrists, forearms, and shoulders.

The Practice While there are *many* ways to approach side plank, this entrance is one that we particularly enjoy because it makes side plank easy to work into a flow, and it encourages us to "push the floor away" and lift up out of our shoulder joints—actions that are particularly important for approaching arm balances.

Begin in downward-facing dog. Either walk your right hand to the center of your mat or keep it where it is (try both ways and see what feels best for you). Shift your weight into your right hand as you roll onto the outer edge of your right foot and stack your left foot on top of your right (or bring it to the floor in front of your right foot, as shown). Keep both feet flexed.

You can place your left hand on your hip or reach your left arm up. Gaze straight ahead or turn your head to look up at your left thumb. Push the floor away with your right hand, lifting your hips high to the sky.

See if you can stay for three to five breaths, then return to downward dog and change sides.

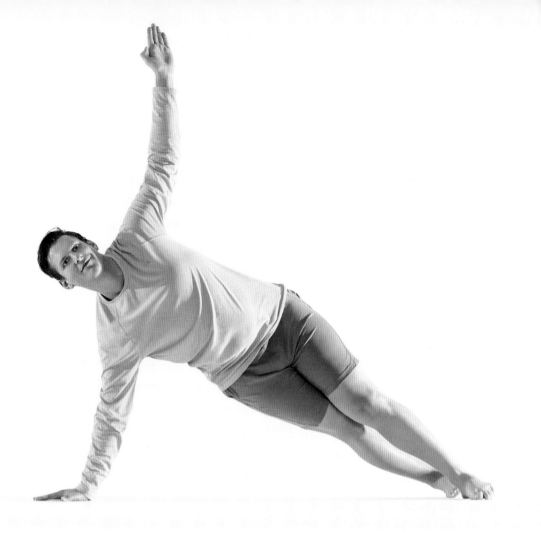

VARIATION 1: FOREARM SIDE PLANK

This is a great variation if you have sensitive or sore wrists. One way to come into it is to begin in a forearm plank (see page 65), stacking your shoulders over your elbows and your heels over the balls of your feet. From here, bring your right forearm parallel to the top of your mat, keeping your elbow under your shoulder. Roll onto the outer edge of your right foot and stack your left leg on top of your right. Keeping your hips lifted, place your left hand on your hip or reach your left arm up. Stay for three to five breaths, then return to forearm plank and change sides.

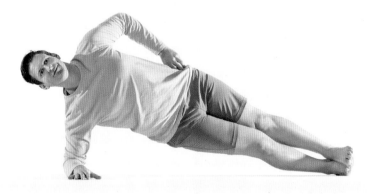

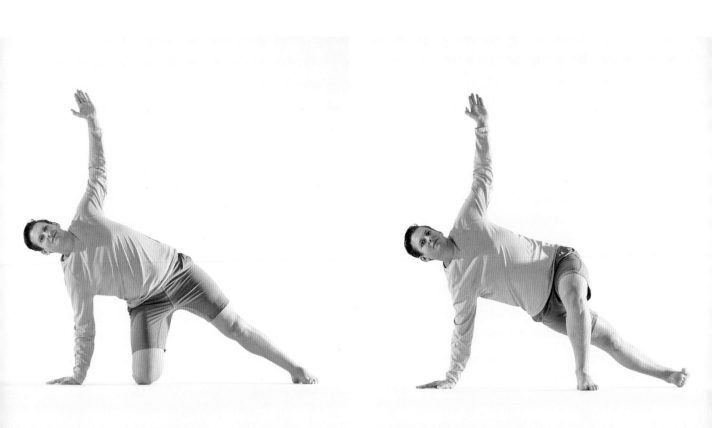

VARIATION 2: KNEELING SIDE PLANK

Begin on hands and knees. Stretch your left leg out long behind you with your left toes tucked under and the ball of your left foot on the floor. From here, shift your weight into your right hand and stack your left hip over your right; pivot and plant your left foot so that the outer edge of the foot is parallel with the back of your mat. Turn your right toes out to the right like a kickstand behind you (this will help with balance), and bring your left hand to your hip, stacking your shoulders and opening your chest to face the left side of your mat. Press down through your right hand as though pushing the floor away. Keep your left hand on your hip, or stretch your left arm up. Gaze forward or up toward your left thumb. Stay three to five breaths, then return to hands and knees and change sides.

VARIATION 3: SIDE PLANK WITH ONE FOOT IN FRONT

This variation can be easier to find your balance in, and it can be fun to work into vinyasa flow transitions. Let creativity be your guide!

Begin in downward dog. Step your left foot halfway up your mat, bending your knee and turning your left foot and leg to face the long left side of the mat. Roll onto the outer edge of your right foot, flexing it, and shift your weight into your right hand. Press down firmly through the outer edge of your right foot, push the floor away with your right hand, and lift your hips high. Bring your left hand onto your left hip, stack your shoulders, and open your chest. Stay here or reach your left arm up. Gaze forward or up. After three to five breaths, return to downward dog and switch sides.

FLYING COMPASS POSE

(Visvamitrasana, Arm Balance Dedicated to Sage Visvamitra)

Though *visvamitrasana* can look intimidating, it becomes more approachable if we break it down into its component parts. For example, instead of looking at it as complicated arm balance, what if you saw it as a variation of side plank? It's sometimes referred to as "flying compass pose" due to its resemblance to revolved sundial/compass pose (see page 117). In that way, it's sort of side-plank/compass-pose mashup! Here, we'll start by exploring a side-plank variation that resembles visvatrasana along with other customizable variations so you can find a version that works for you.

Benefits Due to its complexity, you might think of visvamitrasana as a "whole body" pose that allows you to integrate many different aspects of yoga practice: arm balancing, side-body stretching, shoulder opening, and hamstring opening—to name a few!

The Practice Because there's a lot going on in this pose, we suggest approaching it progressively, step-by-step, which is why we've included variations that break down the key components of visvamitrasana before the more "traditional" form of the pose.

VARIATION 1: ROCK STAR

Also known as "fallen-triangle pose," rock star is a great preparation for, or alternative to, visvamitrasana. Begin in downward dog, and on an inhale, lift your right leg in the air (a position often referred to as "three-legged dog"). On an exhale, bend your right knee and bring it across your body, toward your left upper arm. Keep your right knee there and spin your left foot to the floor, heel pointing to the right and toes to the left. Bring your left hand to your right shin, below your knee, and draw it closer into your chest. You can stay here or try to keep your right knee where it is as you let go of it.

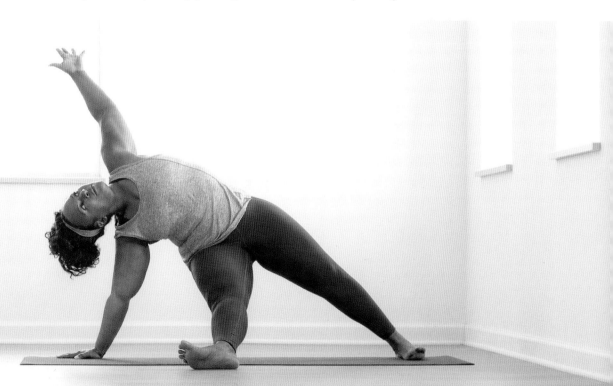

Keep your right knee bent, or kick your right foot straight out to the left, flexing your right foot and keeping your leg lifted high, perhaps stretching your left arm straight up to the sky. Lower the pinky-toe edge of your right foot to the floor, keeping your right foot as close to the top of your mat as possible. Gaze down, forward, or up depending on what feels best for your neck. Enjoy a few breaths here.

To come out, you can plant your left hand and return to downward dog, or you can slide your legs apart from each other to lower your seat to the floor, ending in a wide-legged seated position. Either way, do both sides.

VARIATION 2: ROCK STAR WITH A KICK!

If you'd like to add in a little more strength building or balance challenge, instead of lowering the pinky-toe edge of your right foot to the floor, keep your right leg lifted. Stay for a few breaths, then plant your hand to return to downward dog, and switch sides.

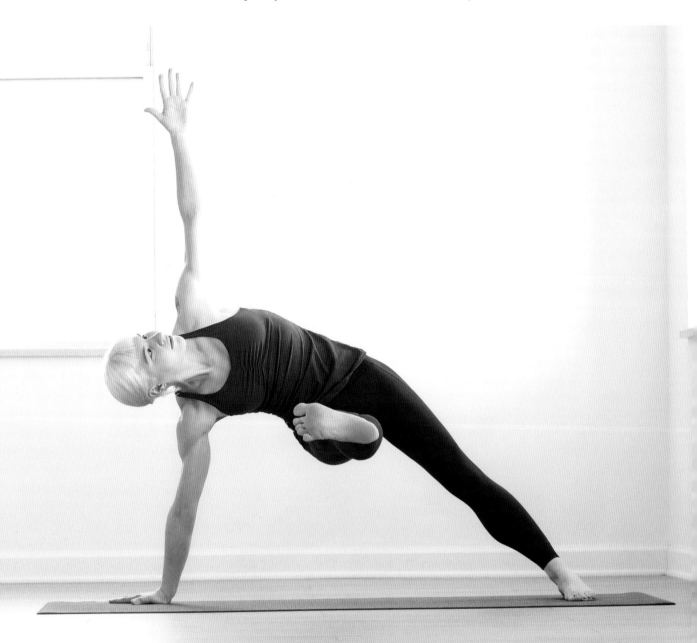

VARIATION 3: VISVAMITRASANA WITHOUT SHOULDER BIND

In the "traditional" form of visvamitrasana (which we'll unpack soon) you work the shoulder/upper arm of your supporting arm under your front leg—a feat that can be challenging even if you're *not* arm balancing! Removing this element can make the pose more accessible.

For this variation, you'll set up like rock star with a kick, stopping at the point where you draw your bent right knee into your chest. From there, keeping your right knee where it is, catch hold of the pinky-toe side of your right foot with your left hand. You can stay here, or, straighten your right leg straight out to the left (like rock star with a kick, but holding your foot).

You can stay there, or sweep your leg forward so that your right foot is pointing toward the top of your mat and your right leg and right upper arm are pressing into each other. Spin your chest up and look up, if that feels comfortable for your neck. Stay for a few breaths, release your foot, and return to downward dog when you're done, then switch sides.

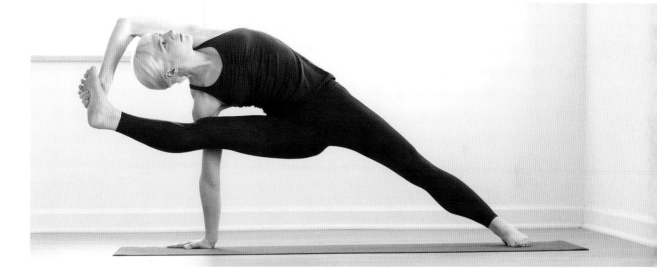

VARIATION 4: KNEELING VISVAMITRASANA

This variation brings the shoulder bind into the mix, but from a kneeling position, which is closer to the ground than the other variations and may feel a little more stable.

Begin in a low lunge with your right foot forward and left knee down, left toes tucked under. Bring both hands to the inside of your right foot. From here, pivot your left toes to the right, bringing your left shin to something of a forty-five-degree angle to create a "kickstand" to help with balance.

Begin to work your right shoulder/upper arm under your left leg: bring your right hand to your right calf and lift the flesh of the calf up toward your knee. Keeping that, move your right thigh back (stick your butt out to the right), which will make space for you to get your leg up over your arm. Continue to work these three actions:

1. Calf up

2. Thigh back

3. Shoulder under, until your shoulder is as "under" as it can get.

TIP If you feel stuck, try lifting your right heel away from the floor as you do these actions to make more space. Then lower your heel toward the floor when your shoulder is as under as it can be.

Next, plant your right hand flat on the floor outside your foot. Press your right leg into your arm and press your arm back into your leg. Then, bring your left hand to your left hip and see if you can lift your right foot away from the floor without using your hand. If you were able to lift your foot, hold on to the pinky-toe edge with your left hand. Remain here or, keeping your arm/leg connection, begin to straighten your right leg. Roll your right hip under and spin your chest up. Gaze up if it's comfortable. When your exploration is complete, bend your right knee and return to low lunge. Then switch sides.

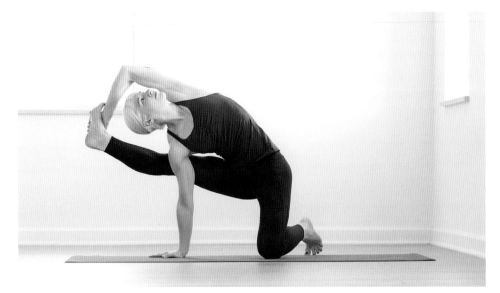

VARIATION 5: STRAIGHT BACK LEG WITH A SHOULDER BIND

This is considered the "traditional" form of the pose, but that doesn't make it better, or even harder than the other variations; it just makes it the variation that's most commonly depicted.

Begin in a lunge with your right foot forward and back (left) leg straight. Spin your back foot down into a warrior II position (see page 72). From here, work your right upper arm/shoulder under your right leg as described in the previous variation, using the three-step process of lifting the flesh of your calf, moving your thigh back, and working your shoulder under until it's as under as it can be.

Then, plant your right hand on the floor outside your right foot. Press your right leg against your arm and your arm against your leg. Bring your left hand to your hip and lift your right foot off the floor without using your hand. If your foot is up, catch hold of the pinky-toe side with your left hand. Stay here, or, begin to straighten your right leg, keeping your arm-leg connection as you do. Roll your right hip under and spin your chest up. Gaze straight ahead or look up.

To come out, bend your front knee and return to a lunge. Then switch sides!

CROW POSE (Kakasana)

Crow is one of the first arm balances that yoga students learn. When practiced with straight arms, it's known as *bakasana* (crane pose), though colloquially the terms *kakasana* and *bakasana* and crow and crane tend to be used interchangeably.

Crow pose requires a great deal of courage, balance, and core strength. To make it more accessible, you can try variations using a variety of props. One caveat to keep in mind: Because your arms are pinned under your knees there is a chance of falling on your face. This unfortunate outcome often keeps students from trying this pose. We tell our students to try this pose outside on the grass to begin or to place a bolster or stack of blankets in front of them to serve as a "crash pad" just in case, and to try to channel their fearless eight-year-old self in order to make crow a little less scary!

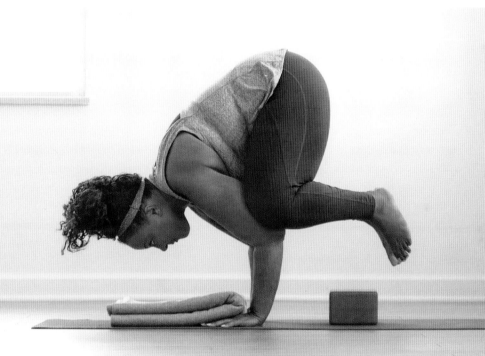

Benefits Kakasana helps strengthen the wrists and arms while also increasing flexibility in the spine by stretching the upper back muscles. Maintaining balance in this pose requires core strength. Regular practice may also build focus and concentration.

The Practice Begin in a deep squat with your feet mat-width apart and your bottom as close to the floor as possible. Bring your elbows inside your knees with your upper arms pressing into your thighs. Try to get your knees as close to your armpits as possible. Then, place your hands flat on the floor in front of your feet, about shoulder-width apart, fingers spread comfortably. As you bend your elbows outward, press your knees inward. Rise on your toes and lean forward, looking straight ahead. Begin transferring your body weight into your arms. Lift one foot, and then the other. Squeeze the inner edges of your feet together. Push your hands into the floor as though pushing it away from you. Once you find your balance in this pose, keep your gaze straight ahead as opposed to looking back toward your feet. This will help you to maintain your balance. Stay a few breaths then return your feet to the floor.

Some people prefer to practice crow pose with their knees outside of their elbows/ upper arms, using the resistance of the legs pressing against the arms and the arms pressing against the legs for stability. Others prefer to have their knees more on the back of their upper arms. Try it both ways and see what works for you.

TIP You can try coming into the pose from a block, to give you a higher starting place for easier access (as Dianne shows in the photo). Start standing on a sturdy block in a wide-knee squat. Hug your knees into your arms as you plant your hands on the floor in front of you, shoulder-width apart. Follow the directions above.

VARIATION 1: RECLINED CROW

This is a great variation if you want to avoid bearing weight through your hands and wrists. It also eliminates the risk of falling on your face completely, and it's a great way to familiarize yourself with the shape of crow pose if you'd like to build up to the arm balance.

Begin on your back with your knees bent and feet flat on the floor. Bring your knees into your chest. Spread your knees wide and bring your elbows to the inside of your knees. Press your knees into your elbows, and your elbows into your knees. Press your palms up to the sky as if you are pressing into the ceiling. Engage your core by drawing your low ribs toward your hips and pressing your lower back toward the floor. You can keep your head down or lift it up. Stay for a few breaths, then release.

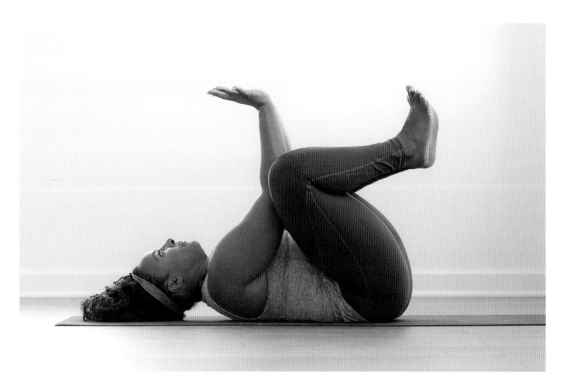

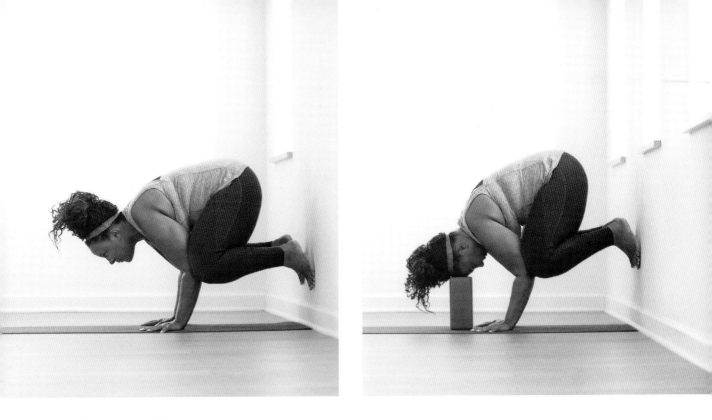

VARIATION 2: AT THE WALL

Try this variation if you find it challenging to keep your feet off the floor in crow. Stand with your back facing the wall, a few inches away from it (as with all arm balances at the wall, you may need to adjust your distance as you go in order to customize the pose to your proportions). Set up as you would for traditional crow. As you begin to transfer your weight into your hands, lift one foot and place it on the wall, then bring the other foot to meet it. Press your hands into the floor while pressing your feet into the wall. Continue to gaze forward. Stay for three to five breaths if possible, then lower one foot at a time to come out.

You can also try this variation with a block under your forehead for more balance support (as Dianne shows in the photo). When you set up, place a block in front of you, on its tallest horizontal setting. Press your forehead into the block as you begin to lift your feet to the wall. If you feel stable, lift your forehead away from the block. Stay here for three to five breaths. If your forehead is on the block, lift it away to come out and return one foot at a time to the floor.

SIDE CRANE/CROW POSE (Parsva Bakasana)

Many of our students have told us that side crow was easier for them to learn than crow pose. Nonetheless, side crow requires a great deal of core strength and a great deal of courage. Though it needs a good amount of physical preparation, the most important skills for practicing side crow are focus and determination.

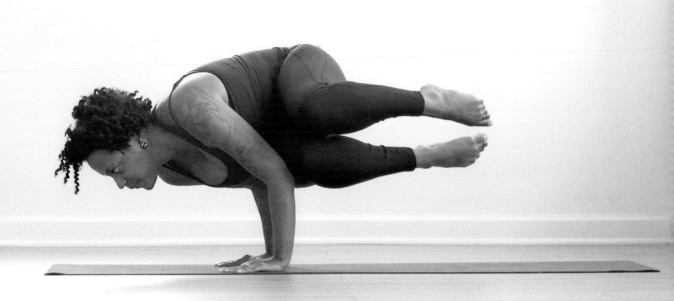

Benefits Side crow offers an excellent strength challenge for your shoulders, arms, and wrists. It also requires a big twist, which activates your obliques.

The Practice Begin standing at the top of your mat in chair pose with legs together (page 44) Bring your hands to a prayer position at your heart. With your legs squeezing together, lift up on the balls of your feet and squat down low. Twist your torso as far as you can to the right and hook your left elbow outside your right thigh. Place your hands on the floor, about shoulder-width apart.

To lift into the arm balance, start to lean forward, pressing your outer right thigh into your left upper arm. Bend your elbows as you slowly start to lift your top (left) leg, and see if you are feeling balanced. If you feel confident that you are stable, try bringing your right foot up to meet your left. Even if you are only airborne for a few seconds, keep practicing. Gaze slightly forward on the floor. Stay for a few breaths if you can, then lower down, untwist, and change sides.

VARIATION 1: WITH BLOCKS

Begin in chair pose with your feet together and two blocks side by side (on their medium vertical settings) next to your right ankle. Hug your legs together and bring your hands to prayer at your heart center. With your legs squeezing together, lift up

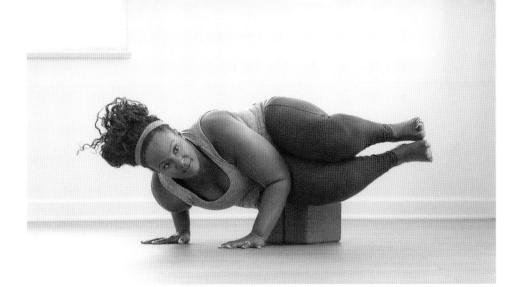

on the balls of your feet and squat low, resting your right hip on the blocks. Twist your torso as far as you can to the left, placing your hands on the floor, shoulder-width apart. With your left elbow pressing into the top of your right thigh and your right hand under your shoulder, float your feet away from the floor. Gaze wherever feels comfortable. Stay here three to five breaths, then release and change sides.

VARIATION 2: AT THE WALL

Stand with your left side a few inches away from the wall and come into a chair pose with your legs together (you may need to adjust your distance from the wall as you go to accommodate your unique proportions). With your legs squeezing together, lift up on the balls of your feet and squat low. Twist your torso as far as you can to the right. Hook your left elbow behind your right thigh. Place your hands on the floor, shoulder-width apart.

Begin to lean forward, shifting more weight into your hands and pressing your outer right thigh into your left upper arm so you can lift your left leg and place the sole of your left foot on the wall. Press into the wall with your left foot, and, once you feel balanced, bring your right foot to meet it. Press your hands into the floor and your feet into the wall. Take your gaze forward past your hands. Stay three to five breaths, then return your feet to the floor, untwist, and change sides.

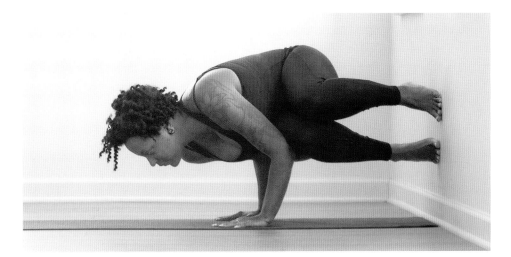

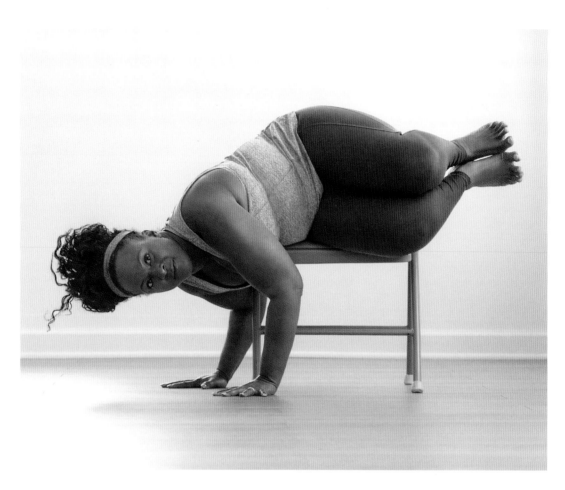

VARIATION 3: WITH A CHAIR

This version of side crow is even more supportive than the wall variation and requires less weight-bearing through your hands and wrists. Sit sideways on a chair with your left side facing the back of the chair, hands at heart center. Lengthen your spine and twist your torso forward to face the front of the chair. Squeeze your legs together and root down into the chair to maintain your balance as you lean forward and place your hands on the floor (or on blocks on their flattest setting) shoulder-width apart, lifting your feet off the floor. Squeeze your knees together and hug them toward your left elbow, balancing your hips on the chair. Take your gaze forward or down between your hands. Stay for three to five breaths, then return to your starting position and turn around so that your right side is facing the back of the chair to change sides.

FLYING PIGEON POSE

(Eka Pada Galavasana, Arm Balance Dedicated to Sage Galava)

Eka pada galavasana is often called "flying pigeon" owing to its resemblance to one-legged king pigeon pose (see page 111). We think this is a particularly fun pose to explore with props, which reminds us that the simple addition of blocks or the wall—or both—can make a big difference!

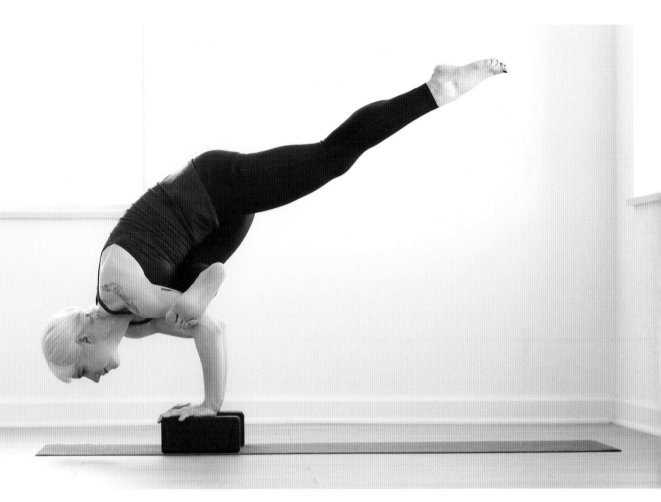

Benefits This pose requires, and over time can build, a good amount of shoulder and core stability. While the earthbound version of one-legged king pigeon offers a feel-good hip stretch (for some), this pose offers an exhilarating arm balance that we highly recommend!

The Practice Here, we'll explore eka pada galavasana with blocks under the hands; however, you're welcome to practice it with your hands on the floor instead. We like the blocks because not only do they make the pose more accessible if your hips are on the tighter side, they also make it easier to keep chaturanga alignment—preventing your shoulders from dipping below your elbows, thus giving you a more stable foundation.

Start by standing at the top of your mat with your feet hip-distance apart and your blocks lengthwise and on their flattest setting, a few inches in front of your toes. From here, come into standing figure-four position: bring your hands to your hips, cross your right ankle over your left thigh, flexing your right foot, and sit back to come into a one-legged chair pose. Bring your hands to your heart, or wherever feels best.

Stay here and enjoy the balance challenge and/or hip stretch, or, if you're ready to explore the arm balance, with a long spine, begin to hinge forward at your hips, sitting back deeper and placing your hands on the blocks, shoulder-width apart. Place your hands near the top of the blocks, gripping the top and sides with your fingers and thumbs if you like.

Hook your right toes as high up around your left upper arm as you can, and lean forward to press your right shin into your right upper arm. Gaze forward and shift your weight forward, bringing more weight into your fingertips and rising high onto the ball of your left foot. See if you can squeeze your left heel in toward your seat, lifting the foot from the floor. Press down into the blocks as though you're pushing them away from you. Keep your shoulders higher than your elbows.

Stay here, or see if you can extend your left leg back behind you.

Aim to stay three breaths (or longer) and then exit the pose with as much control as you used to enter it. Re-bend your left knee and place your left foot on the floor. Return to standing figure four, then back to standing on two feet. Switch sides.

TIP If you're concerned about face planting, place a bolster or stack of folded blankets in front of you to serve as a crash pad just in case.

VARIATION 1: AT THE WALL

This is a great variation to try if you're having difficulty lifting your bottom foot from the floor, or if you just want to have fun climbing up the wall!

Bring the short edge of your mat to the wall. Stand facing away from the wall, close enough that your butt will almost touch it when you sit back in standing figure-four pose. If using blocks, place them on their long flat setting a few inches in front of your toes.

Assume your standing figure-four pose with your right leg on top and hinge forward, placing your hands on the blocks (your butt will likely touch the wall as you do). Wrap your right foot as high up around your upper left arm as you can and press your right shin into your right upper arm. (You'll shift forward to do this, and your butt will probably move away from the wall.) Gaze slightly forward and, keeping your right foot hooked around your left upper arm, shift forward, coming onto the ball of your left foot. From here, hop your left foot onto the wall as close to hip height as possible. (This is easier if you don't think about it too hard!)

Press your hands into your blocks and keep your shoulders higher than your elbows. Keep your left foot on the wall or play with shifting your weight forward more to lift your toes away from the wall.

When your exploration is complete, return to standing figure four and switch sides.

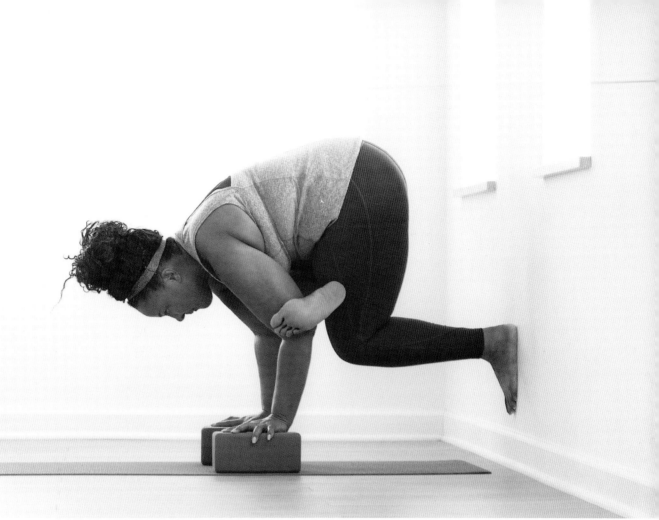

TIP If your right foot starts sliding down your left arm quite a bit, try coming out of the pose and moving closer to the wall.

If you'd like to work on extending your back leg while continuing to work at the wall, you can set up farther away from the wall. Your ideal distance from the wall will depend on your proportions, and finding it may take some trial and error. For a good starting place, measure your leg's length away from the wall and set your blocks on their flat vertical setting so that their near ends are a bit behind where your heels were. Then, come to standing with your toes about an inch behind your blocks and set up your standing figure four.

Instead of hopping your bottom foot onto the wall, you'll squeeze your heel in toward your seat as you lift your foot away from the ground. From there, you can stretch the leg back behind you and place the entire sole of the foot on the wall.

If you aren't able to straighten your back leg when the sole of your foot is on the wall, or if you feel like you'd face plant if you tried, come out of the pose and set up farther from the wall. If the entire foot doesn't come to the wall, come out of the pose and set up closer to it.

If your hands are too close to your feet, it's difficult to lift your bottom foot off the floor, so if you're not using blocks, make sure to place your hands several inches in front of your feet.

VARIATION 2: FOOT ON BLOCK

This variation gives your bottom foot a literal lift, which can make getting it airborne easier.

Often, the trickiest part of this variation is figuring out how to get your bottom foot on the block! We'll explore two ways to do that, starting on the opposite side this time. (We're big proponents of changing things up and not *always* starting on the same side!)

One way is to hop onto the block. Begin in mountain pose with a block on its lowest setting in front of your right foot (the block can be lengthwise or widthwise). Come into standing figure four with your left ankle over your right thigh. Lean forward and plant your hands, shoulder-width apart or a little wider, at least several inches in front of the block. Then hop your right foot onto the block.

Another way is to begin standing on the block. Place a block on the ground, lengthwise on its lowest setting, and stand on it with your right foot. Cross your left ankle over your right thigh to come into standing figure four. Lean forward and plant your hands on the ground, shoulder-width apart or wider. You might want to hop your right foot back a little so the ball of your foot is centered on the block.

Then, regardless of how you got up onto the block, start to lean forward, coming high onto the ball of your right foot if you're not there already, hooking your left toes around your right upper arm, and pressing your left shin into your left upper arm to lean forward a little more.

You can keep your right toes on the block or shift more weight into your fingertips, maybe lifting your toes off of the block and squeezing your right heel into your seat. Stay there, or experiment with stretching your right leg back behind you. Hold your chosen variation for a few breaths, then return to your starting position with your foot on the block, stand up, and switch sides.

VARIATION 3: SHIN ON A BLOCK

This too is a great variation to work with if lifting your bottom foot is challenging, and it's an excellent "sneaky strength builder"!

Begin in mountain pose with a block just in front of your right foot on its tallest and narrowest setting. Come to standing figure four with your left ankle over your right thigh. Sit your hips back, lean your torso forward, and place your hands on the floor, shoulder-width apart or so, in front of the blocks. Hook your left toes around your right upper arm and press your left shin into your left upper arm. Gaze slightly forward. From here, place your right shin on the block and lift your right foot off the floor.

Press your hands into the floor keep your shoulders higher than your elbows.

Either keep your shin on the block or, as you push the floor away, see if you can hover your right shin off the block, squeezing your heel in toward your seat. If you're able to hover your shin off of the block, you can experiment with stretching your right leg back behind you. When your exploration is complete, return your right shin to the block if it's not there already, come back to standing figure four, then mountain pose, then switch sides.

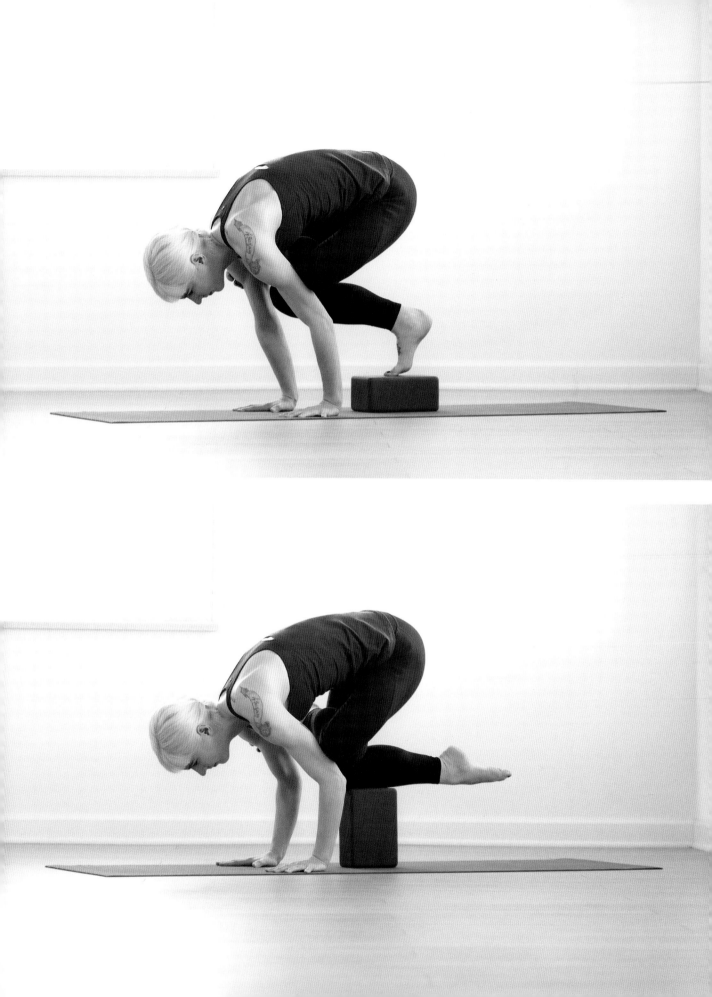

FLYING SPLITS (Eka Pada Koundinyasana II, Arm Balance Dedicated to Sage Koundinya)

We love to explore this arm balance because it's filled with so many possibilities! There are lots of ways to get into it, interesting ways to incorporate props, and it can be fun to include in a vinyasa flow or practice on its own.

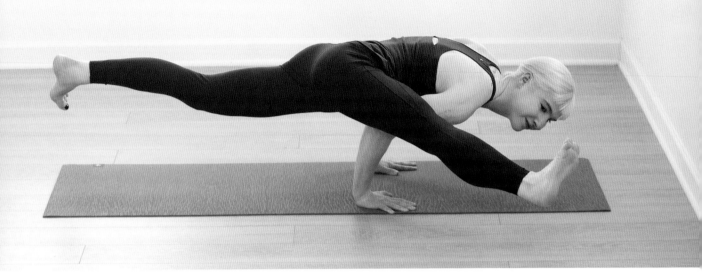

Benefits As an arm balance, flying splits both requires and can help cultivate shoulder and core strength and stability. Most of all we love this pose because it's fun and empowering.

The Practice Let's look at two common ways to get into flying splits.

1. From the ground up

Begin in a lunge with your right foot forward and both hands inside your right foot. You may want to experiment with your foot wider or narrower to see what feels best for you. From here, work your right upper arm/shoulder under your right leg.

To work your leg up over your shoulder: Lift your right heel from the floor, bring your right hand to the back of your calf, and press the flesh of your calf up toward your knee. Then, move your right thigh *back* (stick your butt out to the right), creating space to get your upper arm and shoulder under. Keep working these three actions:

1. Calf up

2. Thigh back

3. Shoulder under until your upper arm/shoulder is as "under" as it's going to get.

Then lower your right heel down, plant your hands on the floor on either side of your right foot with your elbows bent (think "chaturanga arms"). Keep your chest broad, the front of your shoulders lifting away from the floor, and your gaze forward.

Then, start to walk your right foot forward, toward the upper right corner of your mat, perhaps lifting it off the floor entirely.

Keep your left foot on the floor, or shift your weight a little more forward, and try to lift your left toes off the floor. To come out, lower your back foot to the floor, followed by your front foot, and "unwind" your shoulder/upper arm from under your leg. Switch sides when ready.

2. From three-legged dog pose

This variation is a common way to incorporate *eka pada koundinyasana* II into a flow, and some people find it more accessible than the previous method. Try both and see which you like best!

From downward dog, inhale and lift your right leg up in the air for a three-legged dog pose. On an exhale, shift forward, as though you are coming into plank, and bend your right knee, bringing it to the outside of your right upper arm. Bend your elbows (like chaturanga) and shift more weight forward, into your fingertips, as you straighten your right leg. Gaze forward. Keep your left toes on the floor, or, continuing to shift your weight forward, see if you can float your left foot off the ground.

To come out, return your left foot to the floor and stretch your right leg back into three-legged dog. Alternatively, you could come out of the pose by swinging your right leg back behind you to come into a one-legged chaturanga!

VARIATION 1: BACK FOOT ON A BLOCK

Place a block at the back of your mat on its lowest setting. Come into a low lunge with your right foot forward and left knee down with your left toes tucked under on top of the block. Place both hands inside your right foot and work your right shoulder under your right knee (as described in option 1 of the practice). Your inner right thigh will rest on your right upper arm like the arm is a shelf. Hug your left arm into your left rib cage. Lower your chest toward the floor and heel-toe your right foot out to the right until you can lift your right foot off the floor. Keep your chest broad, and press into

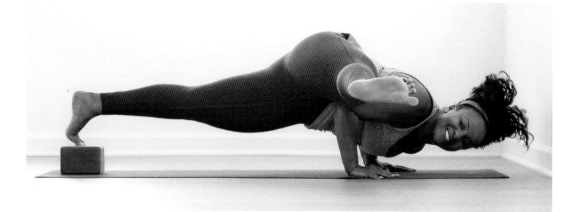

your hands. Press out through your left heel and lift your left knee off the floor. Gaze down toward the floor or look toward your right extended leg. Stay for a few breaths if you can, then lower your left knee to the floor, lower your right foot back to a lunge, and unwind your shoulders. Then switch sides.

VARIATION 2: AT A WALL CORNER WITH A BLOCK

Using a block and two walls can help you support this pose while you're building strength.

Find a corner and start in a low lunge with your right foot forward and left knee down, left toes tucked. One wall should be to your right and the other wall behind you. As you come into the lunge, get close enough to the wall behind you so that the ball of your left foot is on the baseboard. Have a block within reach.

Bring your hands to the inside of your right foot. Have the block in place, on its tallest setting so that it can support your sternum once you've worked your right shoulder/upper arm under your thigh, as described in previous variations. Once you've worked your shoulder under, use the back of your right arm as a shelf for your inner right thigh. Hug your left elbow in, keep your chest broad, and lift your left knee off the floor. Pressing down into your hands, hop your left foot up the wall just above the baseboard. Press down into the block as you heel-toe your right foot out to the side, and then bring the sole of your right foot to the other wall. Push both feet into the walls, press down through your hands, and stay broad though your chest, placing less weight on the block. Gaze slightly forward. Stay for a few breaths, then return to your lunge, unwind your shoulders, and turn around to do the other side.

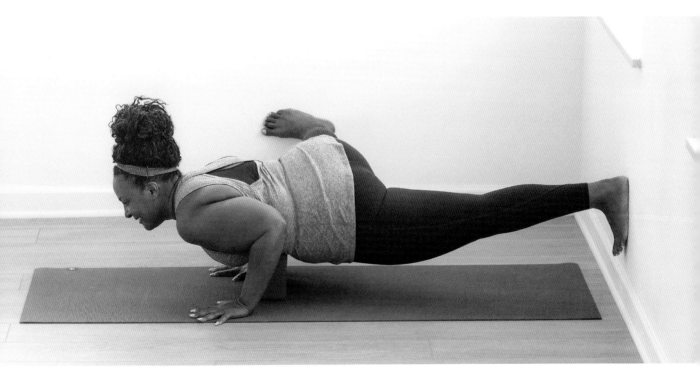

VARIATION 3: FOOT ON WALL, HANDS ON BLOCKS

This is similar to the previous variation, only instead of having both feet on the wall you'll have one foot on the wall. The blocks will give you some extra lift in the pose. Blocks are especially nice if your arms are on the shorter side.

Begin with the short edge of your mat against a wall. Come into a lunge with your right foot forward, facing away from the wall, and the ball of your back foot touching the wall.

Have one block, on its lowest setting underneath each hand. Grasp the edges of your blocks with your fingertips, and think of your blocks as extensions of your hands: they move with you as you work your way into the pose. You can begin with both hands/blocks inside your right foot, but as you weave your right shoulder under your right thigh, your right hand and block will move to the outside of your right foot.

Once your arm is as "under" as it's going to get, with one hand/block on either side of your right foot, bend your elbows for "chaturanga arms" and start to walk your right foot forward, maybe lifting your foot away from the floor. Then, shifting your weight forward into your fingertips a bit more, hop the ball of your left foot onto the wall. Your left knee will be a little bent at first.

From here, straighten your left leg, pressing your whole left foot into the wall. This will shift your weight *more* into your fingertips. Keep your chest and collarbones broad and your gaze forward.

To come out, gently lower your back foot to the ground (bending your left knee a little when you hop down). From there, you can bend your right knee, return your right foot to the floor for a lunge, and unwind out of the pose; or, it might feel good to reach your right leg back, coming into a sweet, spacious downward-facing dog with your heels on the wall and hands on blocks. Switch sides when you're ready.

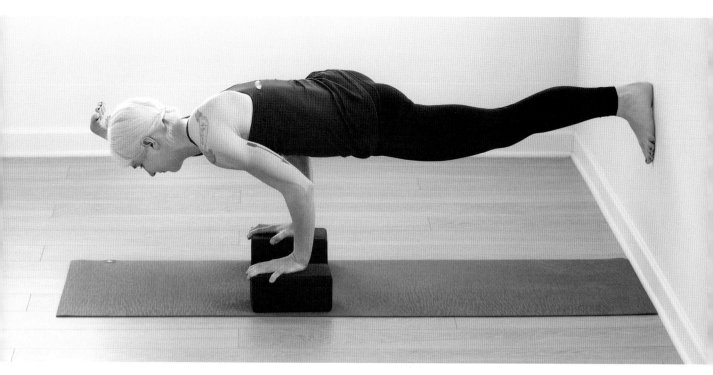

FIREFLY POSE (Tittibhasana)

Firefly derives its name from the fact that your legs in the pose resemble a firefly's antennae. And there's something whimsical about embodying a firefly, isn't there? We encourage you to let this pose's moniker be a reminder to have fun with it!

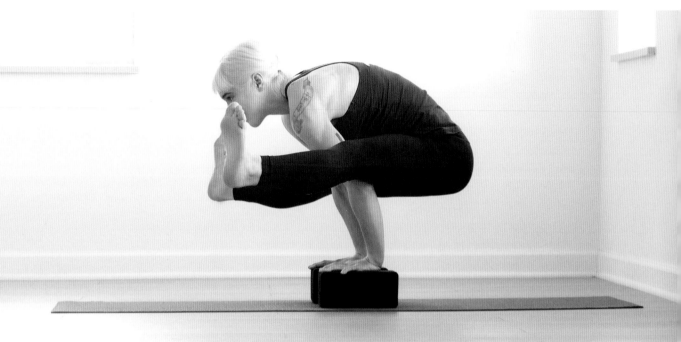

Benefits Firefly pose both requires and can help build upper-body strength.

The Practice Here, we'll explore firefly with blocks. Practicing with blocks under your hands can help you fly a little higher and may make the pose more accessible if your arms are on the shorter side; however, you're welcome to practice with your hands on the floor if you prefer.

To set up, begin in a standing forward bend with your feet wider than hip-width apart and your blocks, on their flattest vertical setting, behind your heels. Bend your knees and, keeping your hips lifted, work your shoulders under your legs: first, lift your right heel up, coming onto the ball of your right foot and, with your right hand, lift the fleshy part of your right calf up toward your knee. Move your right thigh back (sticking your butt out to the right), making space to bring your shoulder under your leg.

Keep working with this three-step process: calf up, thigh back, shoulder under until your upper arm/shoulder is as "under" as it can be.

TIP As you work your right shoulder under, you may want to bring your left hand to your outer right shin pressing your shin in for extra stability.

Then, lower your right heel to the floor and repeat the process on the left side.

Once you've woven your arms under your shoulders on both sides, press your shoulders back against your thighs and place your hands on the blocks (or floor) behind your heels. Grip the front and sides of the blocks with your fingers if you like.

Sit your hips back and bend your elbows straight back so your thighs are sitting on your upper arms. Walk your feet in toward each other. Reach your hips back and your chest forward and see if you can lift your heels so that only the tips of your toes are on the ground.

Press your hands into the blocks (or floor) like you're pushing them away from you, beginning to straighten your arms and round your back, perhaps floating your toes off the floor, straightening your legs. Flex or "floint" your feet. Continue to reach back through your hips and push the floor away.

Stay for a few breaths, then bend your knees, return to standing forward bend, and unwind yourself out of the legs-over-shoulders configuration. Or, alternatively, you might—as gracefully as you can—lower your bottom to the floor to take a seat.

VARIATION 1: AT THE WALL

Stand with your back facing the wall, roughly a foot away from it to begin, with your feet wider than hip-distance apart, and lower your hips to a deep squat, bringing your bottom to rest against the wall. Your elbows will be inside your knees. Press your upper arms against your inner thighs and start to work your upper arms under your legs (your bottom may move away from the wall as you do this). Then place your hands on the floor behind your heels.

Press your bottom against the wall, press your arms into your thighs and your thighs against your arms, and begin to walk your legs out wide in front, straightening them to rest your heels on the floor. You might try to press into the floor and wall and see if you can lift your heels. Gaze slightly forward. Stay for a few breaths, then lower your heels if they're lifted and either return to your squat or lower your seat to the floor to come out.

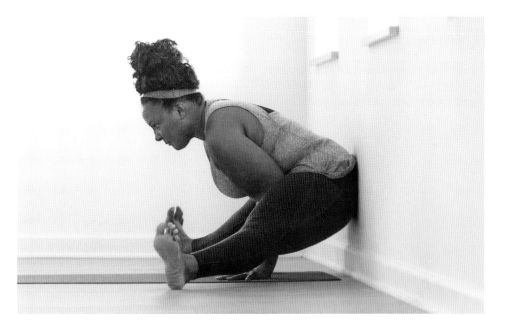

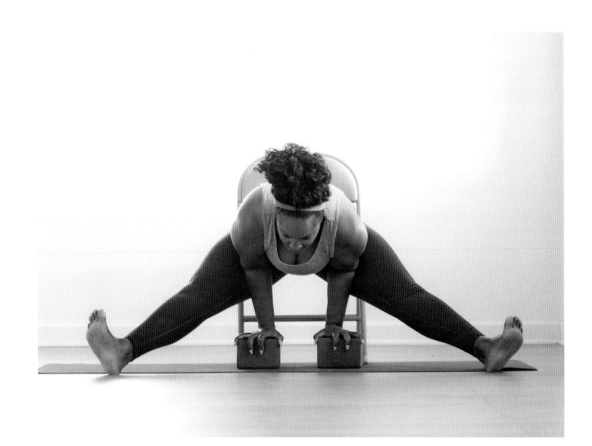

VARIATION 2: WITH A CHAIR

Begin seated in a chair with two blocks on the floor in front of the front chair legs. Have the blocks on their lowest or medium settings and about shoulder-distance apart. Come to the edge of the seat and spread your legs wide apart. From there, lengthen your spine, lean forward from your hips, and place your hands on the blocks, bending your elbows and pressing the backs of your upper arms into your inner thighs. (Make sure your legs are wide enough for you to press the backs of your arms into them.) Walk your legs out to straighten them and press your heels into the mat, flexing your feet. Leaning forward, continue to press your triceps into your thighs and squeeze your thighs into your triceps. Stay for three to five breaths, then bend your knees and return to an upright seat in your chair when you're done.

13

Supine Poses

RECLINED HAND-TO-BIG-TOE POSE
(Supta Padangusthasana)

This classic yoga pose can help make us feel more flexible (in particular our hamstrings!), allowing us to move with more freedom and ease.

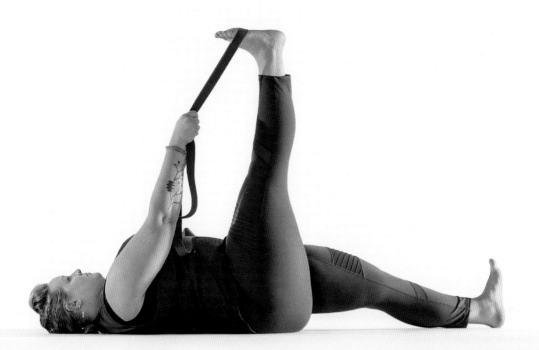

Benefits *Supta padangusthasana* is an excellent stretch for loosening up the legs and creating greater flexibility in the hamstrings.

The Practice Lie on your back and draw your knees into your chest. Extend your left leg long on the floor and keep your right knee hugging in toward you. Make sure that your left toes and knee are pointing up toward the ceiling and that your hips feel level to the floor. Take the peace fingers of your right hand and loop them around your right big toe, or hold on to the pinky-toe edge of your right foot with your right hand, or wrap a strap around the sole of your right foot (as Page shows in the photo).

Straighten your right leg up toward the ceiling, pressing up through your heel as you draw your toes back toward your body. If you're holding your right foot with your hand, rest your left arm next to your body for support or on top of your left thigh to keep the left thigh grounded. If you're using a strap, walk your hands up either side of the strap, as close to your foot as you comfortably can, and allow your shoulder blades to relax down toward the floor. Your arms can be bent or straight.

Stay here for several relaxed breaths, then release your foot from your hand or strap and slowly lower your right leg down to the floor beside your left, reaching out through your right heel as you lower. You might notice that your right leg feels longer than your left at this point! Switch sides to even things out.

VARIATION 1: BOTTOM KNEE BENT

This is an excellent variation if your hamstrings are feeling particularly tight, or if keeping the knees and toes of the bottom leg pointing toward the ceiling feels uncomfortable or inaccessible.

VARIATION 2: STRAP WRAP

Make a super-big loop with your strap (or two straps) and, while still sitting up, bring the loop over your head. Have the strap's buckle in easy reach so you can adjust as needed. Place the back of the loop high up on your back (under your armpits) and lie down on your back. Bend your right knee in toward you, and place the front of the loop over the sole of your right foot. Adjust the tautness of your strap so that when you straighten your right leg the strap holds it in place. You don't need to straighten your right leg all the way. You may also want to slide the back of the loop lower down your back. Take your time to find the position that feels best: where you can lie back and let the strap do its thing.

You can keep your left leg bent or straighten it. Stay several breaths, then bend your right knee to remove your right foot from the loop and change sides.

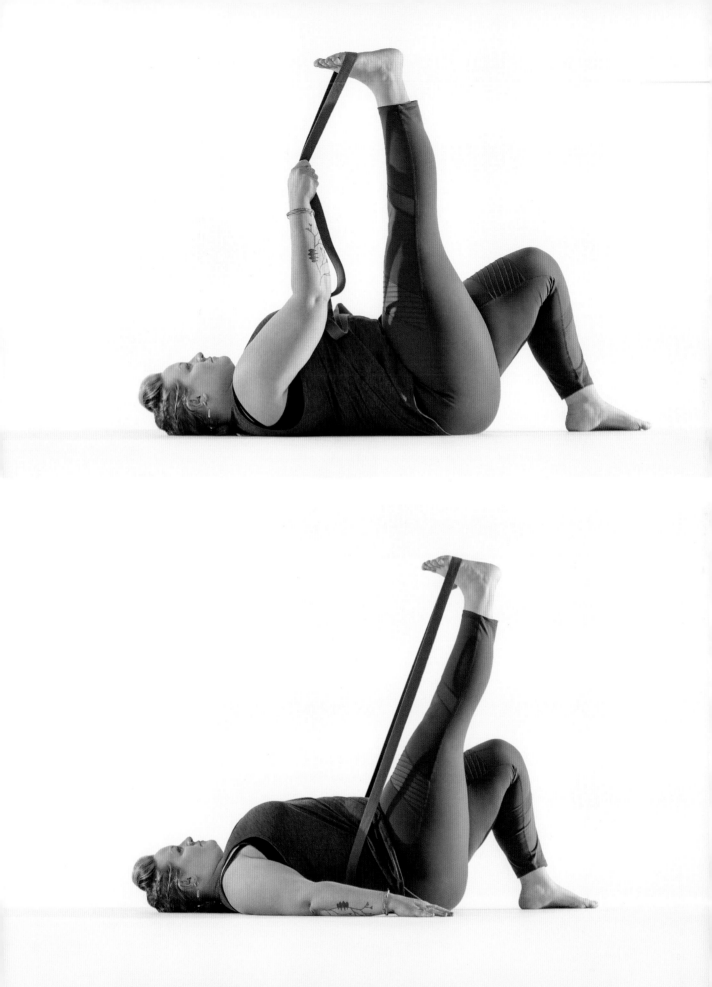

REVOLVED-RECLINED HAND-TO-BIG-TOE POSE

(Parivritta Supta Padangusthasana)

Like *supta padangusthasana* (reclined hand-to-big-toe pose), *parivritta supta padan-gusthasana* (revolved-reclined hand-to-big-toe pose) is an excellent stretch for your hamstrings. Adding a twist can give a little more intensity to the pose and/or change up where and how you experience the stretch.

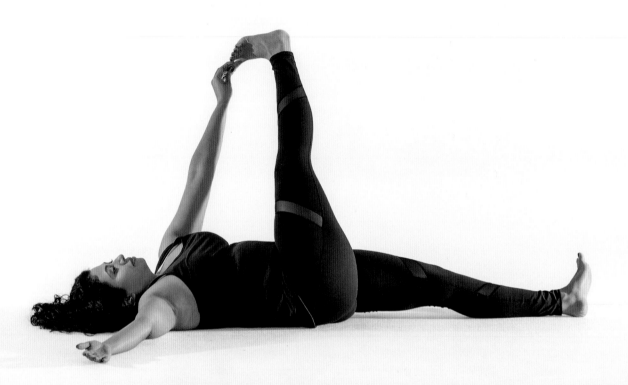

Benefits Revolved-reclined hand-to-big-toe pose can provide a great stretch for the hips, hamstrings, and the IT band.

The Practice Begin by lying on your back with your knees pulled into your chest. Plant your left foot on the mat with your knee bent. With your right knee still hugging in toward your chest, grab hold of the big toe or outer edge of your right foot with your left hand (or use a strap to hold your foot). You can keep your left knee bent or extend your left leg long on the floor with your left toes and kneecap pointing up toward the ceiling.

On an inhale, begin to straighten your right knee, pressing your right heel up toward the sky. Then, still lengthening through your right leg, begin to cross the right leg over toward the left. Stop when you feel a good stretch, perhaps through your outer right thigh. Your left leg may roll open to the left a little as you do this, which is fine as long as it feels good in your body. Extend your right arm out long on the floor at about shoulder height, palm up or down. Keep your gaze upward.

Stay for several breaths, then inhale and bring your right leg back to vertical before lowering it back to the floor. Switch sides.

VARIATION: WITH A STRAP AND BOLSTER

Using a bolster and a strap can help you deepen the twist by supporting your extended leg. Start by lying on your back with your legs long and a large bolster next to your left thigh. Bend your right knee in toward your chest and loop a strap around your right foot. Flex your left foot, keeping your knee and toes pointing upward toward the sky to begin.

Hold the strap in your left hand as close to your foot as possible. Lengthen through your right leg (don't worry if it doesn't straighten completely). Extend your right arm out at shoulder height. Now, cross your right leg toward the left side of your body, resting your right foot on the bolster. Work at keeping your right shoulder anchored to the ground. Remain here for several breaths, and then inhale, to return your right leg to vertical before releasing your right leg from the strap, lowering your right leg to the floor, and switching sides.

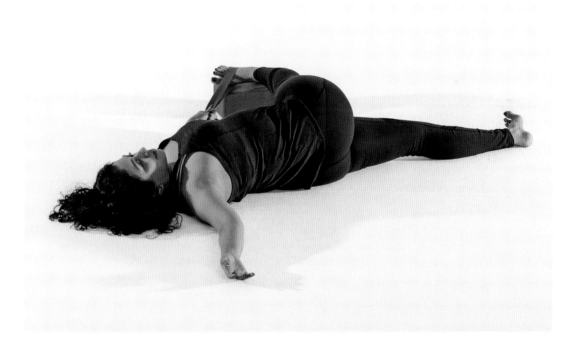

RECLINED TWIST (Jathara Parivritti)

Jathara parivritti (whose name translates to "revolved abdominal pose") is a popular finishing pose in many yoga classes and can be more accessible than seated or standing twists thanks to the support of the floor.

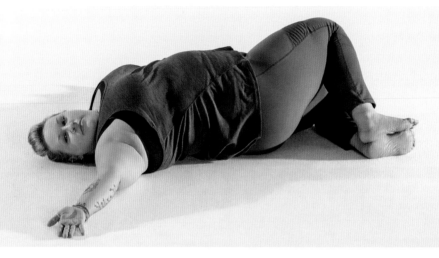

Benefits Many people find supine twists to be relaxing "feel-good" poses. We think this pose feels really wonderful after backbends and hip-opening poses in particular.

The Practice Begin by lying on your back with your knees into your chest. Stretch your arms out to your sides at shoulder level, with your palms up or down. Inhale, then as you exhale bring your knees across your body to the left, lowering them onto the floor. You can gaze up toward the ceiling or turn your head to the right or to the left. Experiment and see what feels best. With each exhalation, twist your belly to the left, away from your knees. Stay for three to five breaths, then return to center on an inhale and switch sides.

TIP If the abovementioned way of getting into the pose feels awkward or uncomfortable, try this: Begin on your back with your feet flat on the floor. Press into your feet, lift your hips up so that you can scoot them to the right and lower them back down. Then lower your knees to the left and continue into the twist from there.

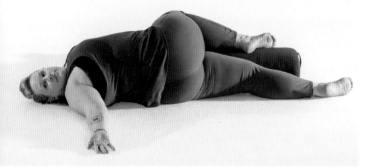

VARIATION: WITH A BOLSTER OR BLANKET

Adding a bolster creates a more restorative version of the twist. One way to use a bolster is to rest your top leg on it for support while extending your bottom leg long (as Page demonstrates in the photo). Or, if there is a lot of space between your knees, place the bolster (or a blanket) between your knees for additional support.

RECLINED BABY CRADLE POSE (Supta Hindolasana)

Reclined baby cradle variations can feel especially good after a leg workout, a standing-pose heavy asana practice, or right before bed. There are lots of ways to dial this pose up or down to make it just right for what you need in the moment.

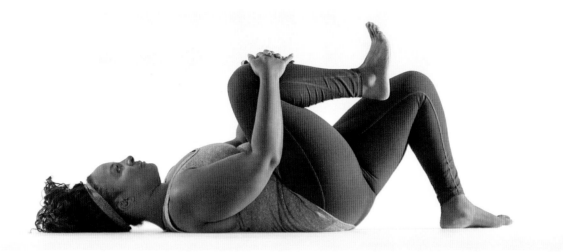

Benefits This pose can provide a feel-good stretch for your outer hips, hamstrings, inner thighs, and lower back.

The Practice Begin by lying on your back with your knees bent and feet flat on the floor. Bend your right knee into your chest, holding on to your shin or the back of your right thigh (you can also hold your thigh with a strap). Draw your knee into your chest and enjoy a few breaths here. See how it feels to bring your right knee toward your right armpit, more toward the outside of your ribcage. If it feels good, stay for a few breaths. You can keep your left knee bent with your foot on the floor, or extend it with your knee and toes pointing up toward the ceiling (as Dianne shows in the photo), depending on what feels best to you. Switch sides when you're done.

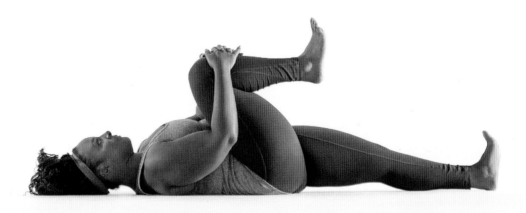

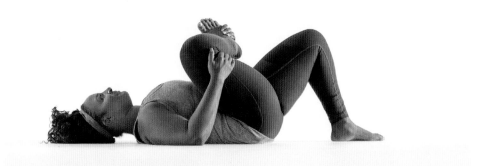

VARIATION 1: BABY CRADLE HOLD

If you'd like to experience more stretch in your outer hip, you can come into a figure four stretch by crossing your right ankle over your left thigh (with your left knee bent, left foot on the floor). Stay here, or to intensify the stretch, draw your left knee into your chest, holding your left shin or thigh. To intensify the stretch further, try a baby cradle hold, holding your right foot with your left hand and your right thigh (below the knee) with your right hand (as Dianne shows in the photo).

Whichever option you choose, keep your right foot flexed and your right ankle straight. Press your sitting bones toward the floor and draw your right foot toward you and your right knee away from you, making your shin as "straight across" as possible. Stay for a few breaths, then change sides.

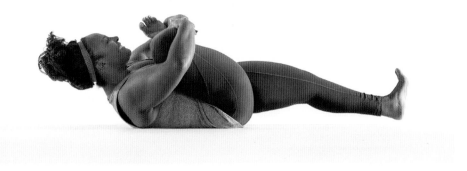

VARIATION 2: ELBOW CRADLE WITH OPTION TO CURL UP

If it's available to you today, you can deepen the cradle hold by bringing your right foot into the crook of your left elbow and your right knee into the crook of your right elbow. Here too, keep your foot flexed and your ankle straight. Draw your right foot toward you and press your right knee away from you. You can keep your left knee bent, or stretch your left leg out long. It's okay if your left heel hovers away from the floor, and it's also okay if it's on the floor. Either way, keep your leg relatively neutral with your knees and toes pointing up. If you like, curl your head and shoulders off the floor. Stay for a few breaths, then release and change sides.

14

Savasana and Alternatives

CORPSE POSE (Savasana)

Ah, *savasana*! The sweet treat at the end of a satisfying practice sometimes referred to as "final relaxation pose." The name technically refers to the pose itself, but sometimes people use it to describe the entire experience of an end-of-class relaxation, which may include silence, music, or guided relaxation. Though savasana is commonly practiced lying on one's back, the important part isn't what the pose looks like, it's that it feels comfortable and relaxing and is a pose you want to stay in for a long while.

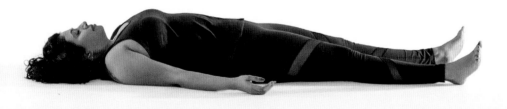

Benefits   When you practice relaxed breathing in savasana, it activates your parasympathetic "rest and digest" nervous system, eliciting the "relaxation response." This allows your body to rest and restore, slowing your heart rate, decreasing blood pressure, and supporting digestion.

The Practice Lie on your back with your legs outstretched. Separate your feet enough so that they can fall open comfortably (heels in, toes out). If you prefer, you can keep your knees bent and feet on the floor. For this option, separate your feet as wide as your mat and allow your knees to drop in toward each other.

Rest your arms alongside you, keeping a comfortable amount of space between your arms and the sides of your body. Turn your palms up, and walk your shoulder blades in toward each other, allowing your chest to be open and broad. Keep your chin level with your forehead (if your chin is lifted, try placing a pillow or folded blanket under your head). You can close your eyes if you like, or keep them open and soft.

Breathe in and out of your nose if possible. Soften your belly so it's free to rise and fall as you breathe.

Often, yoga teachers will say to make your savasana 5–10 percent of your practice: That means, for example, a five- to ten-minute savasana for a sixty-minute yoga class or practice. That can be a helpful guideline to keep in mind when designing a practice, but it's not a hard-and-fast rule. Enjoy savasana as long as you like or can, remembering that even a little bit of rest time can go a long way.

STONEHENGE

There are many ways to customize savasana to make it extra comfortable—for example, with a bolster or rolled-up blanket under your knees. You can also try a Stonehenge setup with a bolster and two blocks.

Prop the bolster up with the blocks. The height of the blocks and how close or far apart they are will depend on how tall/sturdy your bolster is. Experiment, and find a setup that's supportive for you. Lie back with the backs of your knees and calves resting on the bolster, adjusting your position as needed to suit your comfort.

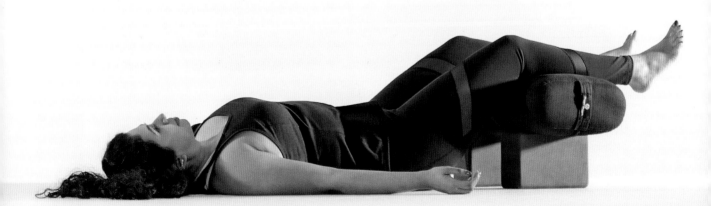

CROCODILE POSE (Makarasana)

Sometimes called "prone savasana," crocodile can be a great alternative if, for any reason, lying face up is uncomfortable.

Lie on your belly. Stack your forearms and rest your forehead on them. Draw your arms in toward you enough that your upper ribs and chest are off the floor (your low ribs stay on the floor).

If stacking your forearms is uncomfortable, you can stack your palms and rest your forehead on the back of your hands. If you do so, walk your elbows back far enough to elevate your upper chest and ribcage away from the floor.

Separate your legs a comfortable distance and turn your toes out. If that doesn't feel comfortable, try bringing your legs closer together and either keeping your feet in a neutral position or turning your toes in.

Soften the muscles of your face, and notice the places in your body that move as you breathe.

Stay as long as you like or as long as you can.

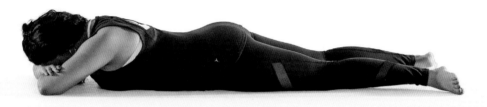

SIDE-LYING SAVASANA

If lying on your back or belly is uncomfortable, you can instead lie on your side. Lie on whichever side you like, though if you're pregnant, lying on your left side is usually recommended.

You can stretch your bottom arm out on the ground and rest the side of your head on your bicep, placing your top arm wherever is comfortable. You could also rest your head on a folded blanket or pillow, resting both arms wherever is comfortable.

Here it can feel great to place a bolster or folded blanket between your knees. You can also place a bolster on the floor behind you for some extra support for your back.

Have your eyes closed or open (remember, that choice is always up to you). Breathe in and out through your nose if you're able. Stay as long as you like or as long as you can.

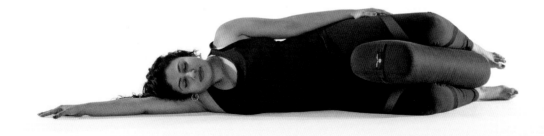

15

Meditation and Compassionate Self-Study

Yoga has touched our lives in ways that go much deeper than the physical poses on the mat. Meditation and compassionate self-study are central to our practice.

Meditation is a practice that helps train one in awareness, learning how to be present without judgment. It's not about becoming better or different, nor is it about how to turn off your brain and stop thinking. Instead, it's about slowing down and turning inward. Meditation, or *dhyana*, is not only part of, but essential to, the yoga tradition.

Meditation can be spiritual—it's an integral part of many religious traditions—or secular. Just as there are many styles of yoga asana, there are many styles of meditation. There are numerous books, apps, and podcasts that can introduce you to the variety of approaches to meditation. We share a couple of our favorite meditation practices after the section on meditation tips.

Numerous scientific studies show the mind and body benefits of meditation, and we've seen this to be true in our own lives through improved focus, confidence, and coping skills. We encourage you to try committing to a regular meditation practice—even just for a few weeks—to see how it might touch your life and your practice.

Compassionate self-study offers a path to meet yourself without judgment, just where you are and just how you are. In this chapter we also share some of our favorite questions for self-study.

TIPS FOR DEVELOPING A REGULAR MEDITATION PRACTICE

Set a goal.

Just as you might when establishing a regular asana practice, try giving yourself a SMART (simple, measurable, attainable, relevant, and time-bound) goal for meditation. This will help you build momentum and to make your practice a habit. For example, your goal might be to meditate for three minutes before bed every day for a month.

Find a style of meditation that works for you.

Meditation styles include, but are not limited to, meditating on the breath, mantra meditation, *metta* or loving-kindness meditation, walking meditation, *yoga nidra* (literally "yogic sleep," a guided relaxation/visualization practice that's often done lying down), and more. If one type of meditation you try doesn't resonate with you, another one may be a better fit.

Choose the right time of day.

The best time to meditate is the time that you're most likely to actually meditate! If you're not an early bird, you might be tempted to skip an early-morning meditation in favor of some extra snooze time, and thus find that practicing during your lunch break or before bed is a better fit. Or you might find that starting your day with meditating sets you up for success and keeps you consistent. If you have a regular asana practice or attend classes consistently, you may try meditating on your mat for a few minutes before or after your practice.

Whatever time you choose, we recommend sticking with it for a set period of time (a few weeks, for example). That doesn't mean you need to be rigid about it, though. If you sleep through your morning meditation on Monday, there's no "rule" that says you can't meditate later in the day instead.

Find a comfortable seat.

It's hard to stick with meditation if it feels painful or uncomfortable! While we often see images of serene yogis meditating in lotus position, the truth is, lotus is not a super-easeful or accessible meditation pose for most people. If you're practicing a seated meditation, your ideal meditation position is comfortable enough that you don't really have to think about it. You can sit cross-legged or kneeling, sitting up on a meditation cushion, yoga block, or folded blanket(s) to help you maintain a long, tall spine. You can also try sitting with your back against a wall and/or placing blankets or blocks under your knees for support if you're sitting cross-legged. Or try meditating sitting tall in a chair. Experiment to find a position that works for you. And if seated meditation isn't your jam, you might find a practice like yoga nidra or a walking meditation is a better fit.

Start small, start simple.

You don't have to meditate for a long time to reap the benefits of meditation. Start with just three minutes. Set a timer. Keep it short. Eventually, you might find that you want to meditate for longer; if so, great! Add another minute or so to your timer. And if meditation starts to feel overwhelming or like a chore, go back to small and simple.

Give yourself a gentle reminder.

Put a reminder in your phone's calendar, pencil *meditation* into your day planner, or try a simple wearable reminder like wearing a bracelet on one wrist before you meditate and then switching it to the other wrist after, or wearing a *mala* (a set of beads often used to keep track of mantra meditations) under your clothing.

MEDITATION PRACTICES

Mantra Meditation

It's often helpful for focus to pair a mantra with the breath. A mantra is a sacred or meaningful sound. In Sanskrit, *man* refers to the mind and *tra* means to "guide" or "protect," so literally, it is a word or sound used to guide your mind as you meditate.

There are many ways to work with mantra in meditation. We'll explore a few of them here.

1. Pair your inhale with a word or quality that you want to "draw in" or cultivate more of, and pair your exhale with a word or quality that you want to share with the world. For example:

> Inhale: Peace
> Exhale: Love
>
> Inhale: Joy
> Exhale: Compassion

2. Pair your inhale and your exhale with an affirmation that's empowering for you. Traditionally speaking, an affirmation is a little different from a mantra, but you can work with an affirmation in a similar way:

> Inhale: I am strong.
> Exhale: I am capable.
>
> Inhale: I am powerful.
> Exhale: I am enough.

3. *Soham* (pronounced *so-hum*) is a Sanskrit mantra that is traditionally paired with the breath and is the first Sanskrit mantra that many meditators learn. It's often

translated as "I am that," and in Vedic philosophy it is understood to connect you with the energy of the universe. It can be coordinated with the breath like this:

Inhale: *so*
Exhale: *ham*

The Practice

Choose a mantra practice that resonates with you. Then find a comfortable meditation seat. Whichever position you choose, sit as tall as you can, aligning the back of your head with the back of your pelvis and lengthening up through the crown of your head.

As mentioned in the "tips" section, we recommend setting a timer for your practice, so you don't have to worry about the time. If you're new to meditation or haven't practiced in a while, try setting it for three minutes to start, gradually lengthening the time you spend in meditation if and as your schedule and interest allow.

Rest your hands wherever they feel comfortable, perhaps on your thighs with your palms facing up or down. Some meditators like to think of palms up as an expression of receptivity and palms down as an expression of grounding.

Close your eyes if that feels comfortable or keep your eyes open and soft.

Begin to notice your breath, breathing in and out through your nose if possible. Allow your upper abdomen and ribcage to expand with each inhale and naturally draw in a little on the exhale. (Your lower abdomen will remain a bit engaged in order to support your sitting upright.) Find an inhalation and an exhalation that are even in both length and quality, one just as important as the other.

Then begin to pair your chosen mantra with your breath.

When you notice your mind wandering, draw your attention back to your breath and your mantra. This is part of the practice, so don't feel as though you're doing it "wrong" if your thoughts stray.

When your timer rings, allow your mantra to fall away, bringing your awareness back to your inhalation and exhalation. Blink your eyes open if they were closed.

If you like, you can rest your hands over your heart or in a prayer position, offering yourself gratitude for taking the time to do something that's good for you or offering gratitude for anything good in your life.

Body Appreciation Meditation

This is a *body reset* meditation, designed to help you reestablish an accepting relationship to your body. Let's move away from our negative programming. We are socialized and trained to view our bodies with negativity and distrust. But this is not who we are. We are not born hating ourselves. A toddler only feels joy and wonder toward their body. Let's return to that time when we blissfully enjoyed our bodies, just as they were.

We've found this meditation practice to help us focus attention on the parts of ourselves that we like—whether physical, emotional, or spiritual—and also to help find an integrated view of ourselves as complex and beautiful humans. We hope it may help you move toward a place of peace with yourself, exactly as you are.

Begin by finding a comfortable position sitting or even lying down. You can close your eyes or keep them softly open.

Now allow your attention to focus on your breath. Watch how the inhalation illuminates the body and how the exhalation enables the body to soften. As you bring your awareness to your breath, begin to notice if your mind is wandering, and if it is, gently bring it back to your breath.

Take a deep breath through your belly and ribs, hold it for a few seconds if that feels comfortable, and then release it slowly. Repeat this action over and over until you begin to feel the body soften.

As you breathe, notice your body rising as your lungs fill with air. Envision your breath as a wave in the ocean. As you exhale, the tide moves out to sea, and as you inhale, the wave rolls back toward the shore.

Imagine that with each wave, that tension in your body begins to release, flowing gently away. Relax your shoulders, relax your jaw, relax the space between your eyebrows. Allow your body to soften into the cushion, chair, or floor.

Say to yourself, *I am here, I am enough, I am safe, I am loved.*

Now, as you continue your deep breathing, shift your awareness to your body. Tap into how your body feels.

As you inhale, take a moment to reflect on all the things your body can do. Notice its ability to love, to feel, and to breathe. Observe how you are feeling in your body. How does your body feel where it touches your clothing? The air?

As you breathe, consider some of the things you are grateful for within your body. You might place your hands on the places you criticize in your body and send them understanding and love. Breathe into those spaces that you are dissatisfied with and send them peace. Tell yourself that it is okay to be here, exactly as you are.

Take some time to consider your own thoughts and ideas about your body. What are you thinking? What do you see? Breathe in . . . and out. As you connect with your body, notice how you are feeling.

Now, imagine yourself making peace with your body as it is. You don't have to love it, but let's set aside anger or hate and look for neutrality. Imagine feeling contentment with exactly where you are at this moment.

What might it be like to feel comfortable with your body? Start to see yourself as a whole divine being with your body as a vehicle to live your life.

What are all the incredible things your body does for you? Think of how it rejuvenates you when you need energy, how it relaxes you when you need rest.

It is okay to be who you are. Repeat. It is okay to be who you are. You are enough.

You might try a new mantra for peace and acceptance. You can repeat all of it as you breathe, or only the lines that most resonate with you.

Breathing in: I am enough.
Breathing out: I do enough.

Breathing in: I have enough.
Breathing out: My body is enough.

Breathing in: My body is a manifestation of my Divine Self.
Breathing out: I am at peace now.

Now, feel yourself on a path of self-acceptance.

When you are ready, begin to awaken by taking deep full breaths and releasing them with a deep sigh. Begin to move your body in a way that feels good to you as you return your attention back to your environment. Slowly open your eyes if they were closed and see the world a little differently.

COMPASSIONATE SELF-STUDY

Just as there are many ways to meditate, there are many ways to practice compassionate self-study. We've found regular journaling to be a powerful practice. We like to use questions or prompts, or you can also free-write.

Journaling doesn't need to take a long time to be powerful. Try writing what comes to mind—even for just two minutes or longer if you're so inspired. There is no need to edit yourself or judge what you write. See what flows. As with meditation, we recommend setting an intention to choose a time of day and making a commitment to try journaling for a set length of time to see what unfolds.

Journal Prompts

» What am I grateful for? (This is a great one to try every day!)

» What is my intention for today? What is my affirmation? (This is a great one to try every day!)

» What am I feeling right now? Is it my breathing, my clothes, my emotions?

» What are my core values? Do my core values align with my actions and feelings around the things I love to do?

» How do my thoughts align with my actions and words?

» What stories am I telling myself? Are they true?

» How will I care for myself today?

» What will I do today that makes me happy?

» What feelings do I want to create in my life? Who will I share them with?

» What do I celebrate about myself right now?

» How is my yoga practice going? How is meditation going? Any reflections or realizations?

» What inspires me?

» What can I release?

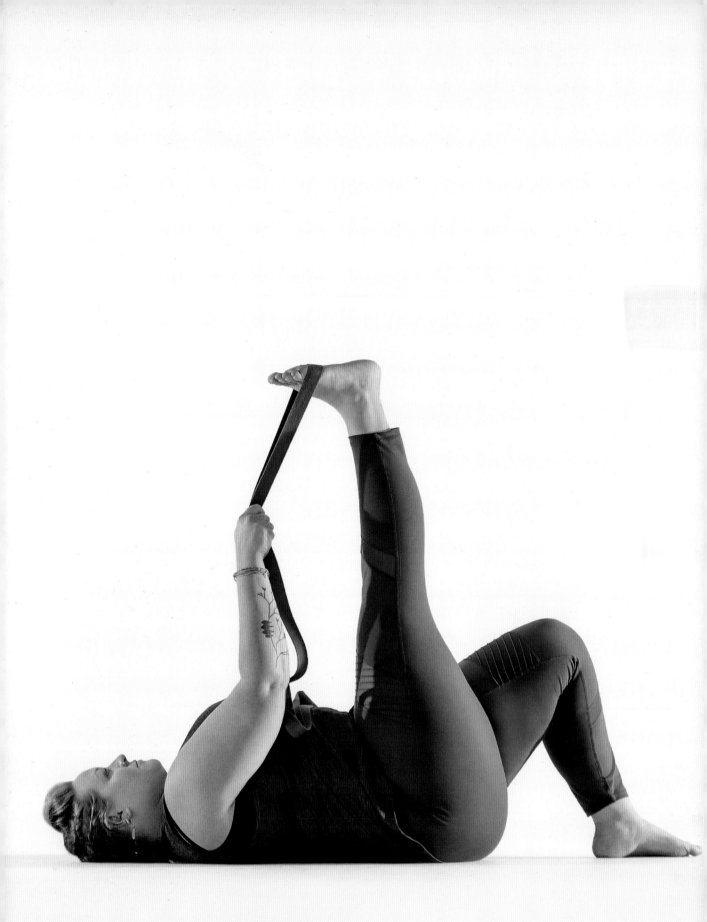

DESIGNING Part Three YOUR PRACTICE

16

Sequencing and Accessibility

Whether we are planning a sequence for personal home practice or to share with students in a class, we like to keep a few key ideas in mind: How we welcome ourselves and our students to the mat matters. The words we use to talk to ourselves and to our students matter. And the practice of yoga can be so much more than just the poses—the opportunities we create for connecting to ourselves, our students, and our world matter.

We hope this chapter will be helpful not only to teachers (and those who train teachers) but also to people aiming to deepen and customize their home practice. First we talk about how we approach our mat, our classes, our students; then how we talk to ourselves and to each other; then we move on to the art of sequencing.

COME AS YOU ARE

Remember that yoga isn't about fixing yourself. It's about being with yourself, and learning about yourself, and that wherever you are today is okay. Your practice grows and changes with you. Just because you could do something yesterday doesn't mean you can, or need to, do it today. And just because you can't do something today doesn't mean you'll never be able to do it again. Every practice and every pose is unique. If this is your first time back to your mat in a while, great! Welcome yourself back. No matter how long a break you've taken from it, yoga is always there for you.

WELCOME YOUR STUDENTS

Creating and holding a safe space for students to enjoy and transform within their yoga practice can be very challenging. Not only are teachers required to make the practice safe physically, but also emotionally. Students with bigger bodies, students who are older, students from diverse backgrounds, students with varying levels of physical ability, and quite frankly, *all students*, can be very self-conscious in a yoga class. Feeling as though you *don't belong* can be scary. This is why the first step is to be welcoming! Greet students, support students, and encourage them to come to class. It is our ability to be welcoming that sets the stage for creating that atmosphere of understanding and appreciation for different body types and abilities in our classes.

Ten Strategies for Creating a Safe Place for All

1. If your goal is to serve a specific population, then develop a class for that population specifically (Yoga for Bigger Bodies, Queer Yoga, Seniors Yoga, etc.). Creating a specialty class may be a way of making sure all students feel seen, included, welcomed, celebrated, represented, and encouraged to practice.

2. Practice *svadhyaya*. Make sure to do your own self-study to identify your own biases around what you believe about bodies different than your own. How might your own personal biases around gender, body size, or ethnicity be impacting your teaching and your students' experiences of yoga? Once you're aware of your biases, what changes will you make to address them?

3. Plan your classes. Come prepared for your yoga class. You have no idea who may show up, and you may need to diverge from your plan, but it is always great to have a plan, and often a theme. It is nice for students to have a message they can take away with them that relates to their lives and invites them into the spirit of "coming to know yourself" through the physical practice. It reminds them that yoga is about more than just the poses.

4. Make sure students feel welcomed—especially new students. Smile and initiate the conversation by introducing yourself. Invite the student into the practice space. Reassure them they have done the right thing just by showing up to class.

5. Learn students' names and show that you care enough to pronounce their names correctly. It is important to your students. It is also important to be aware of, and use, students' pronouns (e.g., her/she, he/him, they/them).

6. Read students' intake forms and be friendly and conversational as you open up the space to discuss any of their challenges or concerns. Remember: always focus on what a student *can do*.

7. Foster connections. You might introduce a new student to one of your regular students or others in the class. Have a regular student grab props for the new student, show them around the studio, or point them in the direction of the washroom. The goal is to create a warm, inviting atmosphere while encouraging students to share their experiences.

8. Never *ever* prejudge students or their situations. Admittedly, this is a hard one. We are all hardwired to judge. So check in with yourself. Figure out what makes you uncomfortable and recognize this experience as a major part of your own practice of teaching yoga. You have no idea what this person is capable of based on their physical appearance. Just because a student might be bigger, older, or different physically, doesn't mean that they can't do the practice.

9. Say what you mean, enunciate your words, speak loudly, clearly, and slowly.

10. Keep instructions simple. We recommend against overly complicating your instructions, and we love allowing some spaciousness in classes for students to be with themselves.

THE POWER OF LANGUAGE AND INTENTION

When thinking about how to welcome yourself or your students to the mat, we encourage you to set the intention to pay careful attention to your language. Honor your body and practice, and honor those of your students.

Yoga teachers commonly use the phrase, "full expression of the pose," to refer to the "classic" or "typical" version of a posture—the one that has been most commonly depicted in photographs. This phrase is very misleading and increasingly archaic. We feel this phrase limits people's view of what a posture should look like within their *own* body. The internal conversation in the mind of the yoga practitioner can transform into one of self-doubt, criticism, and judgment, as thoughts like *I'll never be able to do that* start to creep up. What if we changed our perception to recognize that "the full expression of the pose" is really your very own, uniquely perfect expression of the posture on a given day?

Instead of relying on limited language like "the full expression of the pose," create new phrases like *Come into your individual expression of the pose*. Give yourself or your students the freedom to explore this idea. Encourage students to come to know themselves by choosing positive words like *feel*, *explore*, *engage* in the pose right where you are. Remind them to do what feels good in their bodies.

TIPS

» Watch for gender-specific language, like *ladies and gentlemen*. Use gender-inclusive language such as *folks*, *friends*, *everybody*. When offering modifications for pregnancy, remember that not all pregnant people identify as women. Stay away from stereotypes (e.g., "Women tend to be more intuitive . . ." or "Men tend to be more competitive . . .").

» Describe alternate shapes as pose variations that can offer benefit to anyone, not modifications of lesser value.

» Remember: students can be empowered or devastated by the language we choose to use as teachers. Use invitational language to access the poses instead of commanding your students. When in doubt, err on the side of kindness.

SEQUENCING

There are many different ways to sequence a yoga practice at home or in a class. In this section we'll focus our conversation on yoga teachers, but most of these ideas can apply to a home practice as well.

Some people like to teach on the fly, while others like to plan almost every detail. If you are a yoga teacher, we suggest you come up with a plan of some sort. Planning your class gives you peace of mind, while also allowing you the option of being spontaneous. You appear more professional, confident, and invested in your students' experience.

As teachers, we need to be sensitive to the needs of new students and be open to the desires of our seasoned students as well. Through our classes, we can show people their own power as well as create spaces for self-care, personal growth, and spiritual connection. You can create inspiration and joy by putting together a great sequence with a well-thought-out message. We can change how we move our bodies and connect to our breath. We can even change our consciousness and open our minds to new possibilities.

WHY STUDENTS PRACTICE

We are greatly inspired by yoga teacher Christina Sell, whose work with sequencing is incredible. She categorizes students into three distinct types. This doesn't mean that there are only three types of people who come to the mat, but that many yoga students share common traits that can be useful to consider. Knowing as much as you can about your students' needs, goals, and interests will help you build progressive, accessible, and inclusive classes.

The Mystics want to be inspired. They come for a more spiritual experience of yoga, which might include aspects like dimmed lights, traditional sitar music, and incense. They want a heartfelt experience steeped in yoga philosophy. They come to the mat to seek a sense of peace and connection to a higher power.

The Engineers focus more on the technique of the postures. Engineers are interested in how and why yoga works. They love to learn about not only anatomy, physiology, and biomechanics but also the construction of the practice. You can think of them as the scientists of yoga asana. They want to know the exact angle of the knees and why we do certain asanas. They will come back to class if they learn something.

The Athletes measure the efficiency of class based upon physicality. They come to move, breathe, stretch, and strengthen. And sweat! They like to keep moving and don't want to be stopped for demos. Yoga is part of their physical workout. They enjoy learning a sequence and being left alone to move through that sequence with power.

We'll also add a bonus type: *the Cautious Beginners*. These students are new to yoga. They may have come to the mat because of an injury or a need for stress management. They may have a disability or need greater attention in their asana practice because of trauma, anxiety, or limited physical abilities.

In truth, all students are a combination of all these types and so much more, though we may identify more strongly with one than another. The best way to sequence for your students is to get to know them. Ask questions about their practice, find out what they are curious about. Watch and learn about your students—*that* is the key to being a great teacher.

TYPES OF SEQUENCES

There are many different ways of sequencing a class, depending on what you are comfortable with and what your students' needs are at the time of practice. Be careful, observant, and open to learning. Here are a few examples of how you can sequence a class:

1. Using a set postural sequence, like those taught in Jivamukti, Ashtanga, and Sivananda yoga.

2. Sequencing based on a particular alignment principle, such as those taught in Iyengar yoga.

3. Building toward an "apex" or "peak" pose; for example, sequencing based around a pose such as urdhva dhanurasana (upward bow or wheel pose), determining what other poses you need to do in order to climb the "mountain of a pose," practicing that pose or variations, and then descending the mountain to move toward final relaxation.

4. A potpourri class that has a little bit of everything!

CLASS THEMES

Setting a theme or focus for your class can tell a story and bring an experience full circle. If you'd like to use a theme, here are some suggestions for choosing one:

» Create a theme for a class with music, building a common thread through each song or even craft an entire playlist around an artist whose work inspires you.

» Choose a body part that needs love like shoulders or hips, or even a concept, such as finding balance.

» Have a theme focused on seasonal changes, perhaps rooted in the principles of yoga's "sister science" Ayurveda.

» Devise a theme for your class that is centered around a poem, quote, or short story.

» Create a theme that focuses on a quality or virtue like courage or gratitude.

» A theme can also be an intention such as focusing on your breath, letting go of expectation, or making peace with your body in asana.

KEY CONSIDERATIONS FOR SEQUENCING

» **START WITH A CENTERING PRACTICE** (seated, standing, or lying down). Get students out of their heads and into their bodies.

» **WARM UP.** In a mixed-level class, choose poses that everyone can do fairly easily. Move bigger muscle groups to heat the body.

» **MAKE SURE 80 PERCENT OF THE PEOPLE IN THE CLASS CAN DO ALL OR MOST OF THE POSES IN THE SEQUENCE.** You might have one or two challenging poses that students can work up to or try a variation of, describing all variations as worthy of value. Create stepping-stones or building blocks for the challenging poses that are interesting, accessible, and empowering.

» **COOL DOWN.** Carve out time for students to wind down and prepare for savasana. Include "feel-good poses" that target the areas of the body they worked during class.

» **SAVE TIME FOR SAVASANA.** Plan for at least a few minutes of relaxation. Depending on your teaching style and the interests and needs of your students, savasana could include silence, a guided relaxation practice, or recorded or live music. (For savasana options and variations, see chapter 14.)

BEING BODY-POSITIVE AND HELPING STUDENTS OVERCOME SELF-CONSCIOUSNESS

Many people, including seniors, beginners, people of color, people practicing with disabilities, and people with bigger bodies may feel self-conscious when approaching yoga. In response, teachers need to focus on what students *can* do, rather than on what they *can't* do. By turning awareness back to what *can be done* during the yoga class, and by focusing on the concept of "coming to know thyself," we remind students that they are each their own best yoga teacher. This extends to reminding students that the images they see in the media and the other people they see in the room are not reflections of what *they* can or can't do in their own personal practice.

In order to teach to a diverse group of students, we must attempt to connect with all the individuals in the room, just as they are. Not everyone is going to want to engage in return, but in our experience, if you remain open, honest, and authentic, more and more people will want to practice with you.

CREATING AN INCLUSIVE, ACCESSIBLE, PROGRESSIVE CLASS

As teachers we aim to meet students where they are—but we don't want to leave them there! It is crucial for yoga teachers not to be discouraged by a student with a physical challenge. Instead, we must take these experiences as opportunities to learn more about the practice, our students, and ourselves. We can also keep in mind that public classes don't serve every student well—smaller private or semi-private classes may serve some students better.

Understanding some of the most common challenges facing students in a mixed-level, inclusive yoga class can help us work with students most effectively. These challenges include:

» breasts, butts, thighs, and larger body parts can limit access to certain postures

» self-consciousness and fear of public shaming

» fear of not being able to get into the postures

» judgments about a student's level of ability (from themselves, from other students, and from the teacher)

» inappropriate comments about gender and culture, including gender-specific cues

» music (swearing, inappropriate cultural references, or sexist language)

Overcoming these challenges requires you to use your yoga practice to become a more conscious teacher. Look at your students and pay attention to what you are asking them to do and how you are asking them to do it. Put yourself in the place of the student. Recognize experiences that differ from your own as real and valid. It is easy to default into "teacher mode" or to click into autopilot. Getting grounded and being present yourself will help you be the best teacher for your students.

Here are our top three tips for great teaching at any level:

1. FOCUS ON YOUR STUDENTS

2. BE COMPASSIONATE

3. REMAIN CONSCIOUS OF YOUR LANGUAGE

THE POWER OF PROPS

Props can be used to support and deepen the practice for *all* students. Props can make the difference between classes that are *exclusive* versus classes that are *inclusive*. We discuss props in depth in chapter 5. Teach your class to embrace props as aids that can help them to access a posture, support their body, and ultimately improve their well-being throughout the duration of a yoga class. You will be astounded by how expansive and inclusive your asana class will become with the props—especially in meeting the needs of different body types.

Here are our top tips to unleash the power of props:

1. Introduce and normalize the use of props. Have everyone grab props prior to the start of class—even if students think they may not need them. Then, ask

students to try poses with props to see how they feel in their practice. Let your class know that props are enhancements and not "crutches."

2. Teach your students how to use a variety of props so that they'll feel confident using them in other classes or at home.

3. Experiment with new and innovative ways of using props with your own body as you plan your classes.

4. Teach the "modified version" of the pose using the prop *first*. This normalizes the use of props and doesn't single anyone out.

TRANSITIONS

Beginners, older students, and students with bigger bodies may have trouble with the constant "ups" and "downs" of the yoga practice. Minimizing these transitions within your classes can help make the class more accessible and comfortable for everybody.

One of the hardest transitions for bigger-bodied and new students is the "step-through" transition in which students move into a lunge or standing posture by stepping their foot forward between their hands, commonly from downward-facing dog. Students with tight hips and/or larger bellies, thighs, or breasts will often experience trouble executing this transition smoothly. The best solution here is to utilize the "step-back" method, by giving students the option to begin in a forward fold, and then step one foot *back* to come into a posture instead of stepping a foot forward from downward dog.

Building from the "step-back" transition method, you can move into a wide-legged forward fold, by turning the toes to face the long edge of the mat. This gives the teacher and student the opportunity to transition to lateral-facing poses (such as warrior II, side angle, triangle, and half moon) from a solid, accessible platform.

We share more information on working with students on the "step-through from downward dog" transition in our pose description of downward dog on page 62.

PROGRESSIVE CLASS SEQUENCING

The Bus Stop Method—Slow and Steady Wins the Race

We love Christina Sell's "bus stop method" of sequencing, which is a great strategy for making your classes more accessible.

First, choose the posture you want to teach and practice it in your own body. Take a moment to look at the shape of the posture, consider what other postures share similar shapes, and then group the postures together.

The Bus Stop Method in Action

1. Start at the basic form of the pose and work your way to the final destination.

2. Invite your students to "get on the bus" at the first stop.

3. As the pose builds and becomes more complex, offer the students the opportunity to get off the bus at different stops before arriving at their destination.

4. Remind students to *slow down and enjoy the ride*!

An Example of the Bus Stop Method

» **BUS STOP 1**: Balancing on one leg, drawing the opposite knee into chest.

» **BUS STOP 2**: Warrior III, or beginning in a forward fold with hands on blocks, stabilize one leg as you lift the other behind you, extending energy out through the heel.

» **BUS STOP 3**: Warrior III with one hand on a block and one arm out to the side, or half moon pose with a block.

TIPS

» Make sure you have two or three variations to offer for each pose. Work out these variations on your mat before you teach them in class. Take the time to break down each pose that you offer.

» Give students permission to get off the bus at any stop.

» Pay attention to all students in the room. Remember: you want to create classes in which 80–90 percent of the postures can be easily and comfortably executed by *all* of your participants.

» For the other 10–20 percent of class, you can incorporate the more challenging postures as an opportunity to teach strategies and tips for safe execution and experimentation. Students are generally open to learning new things in classes, as long as they feel safe and supported.

» Be creative!

SEQUENCING FOR MIXED-LEVEL CLASSES

Though the term *mixed-level class*, is common, it's often a misnomer. What you see in many of today's "mixed-level" or "all-levels" classes are often designed for students at the intermediate level. So how do you teach a true mixed-level class? We recommend breaking down the class into digestible chunks.

1. If you're sequencing toward an apex/peak pose, determine your apex pose first, then begin to investigate postures in the same group (i.e., those that are shaped similarly). Use simple postures from the same group to build a warm-up sequence. Alternatively, you could determine your class theme first, investigate postures that connect with it, and use simple poses to build up to those poses.

2. Start introducing variations for poses in the warm-up. This will introduce students to options that they can later utilize when you arrive at the apex pose.

SAMPLE SEQUENCE PLAN

There are MANY different approaches to sequencing a yoga practice or class. (See page 230 for some "outside of the box" options!) The "right" way is the way that's going to best serve YOU or your yoga students. The sequence grid here is one of our favorites for creating a complete, full-spectrum class. Feel free to use it (or modify it) to create sequences of your own.

Keep in mind: You don't have to do a pose for every category. Skip any that don't fit with your present needs, goals, or intentions for practice.

Centering A sitting or kneeling pose, child's pose, savasana, crocodile pose, or mountain pose with a simple reflection and breath-awareness work.

Warm-up Simple, dynamic movements, preparatory stages of poses—for example, a low lunge if you're going to be doing a high lunge later.

Downward-Facing Dog Include dynamic movements to start, such as pedaling the feet, shifting hips and heels from side to side. Introduce options like bending the knees, placing hands on blocks, or coming to hands and knees in lieu of downward dog.

Sun Salutations Sun salute A, B, or any variation that you like.

Standing Poses Warrior poses, triangle, side angle, half moon, standing balance poses, lunge variations, and so on.

Core Work Planks, boat pose and variations, even exercises borrowed from other styles of movement such as Pilates.

Hip Openers Many arm balances require a fair amount of lateral hip and/or hamstring flexibility (think flying pigeon, flying splits, flying compass, firefly), which is why it's helpful to practice earthbound stretches for these areas first, such as pigeon, fire log, cow face pose, and splits variations.

Arm Balances and Arm-Balancing Inversions All arm balances and inversions like dolphin, forearm balance, handstand, scorpion, and headless headstand. You could also do headstand here.

Quad and Hip-Flexor Stretches Hero pose, reclined hero pose, King Arthur pose. (These will help prepare for the backbends that follow, which require a fair amount of quad and hip-flexor flexibility.)

Backbends Bow, camel, bridge, upward bow, and so on.

Seated and Reclined Twists and Forward Bends Seated forward bend, head-to-knee pose, supine twist, any options and variations that help you move inward and prepare for savasana.

Legs-Up-the-Wall pose Or other restorative poses

Savasana You could remain in a restorative pose for savasana, lie supine, or choose a variation such as crocodile pose or side-lying savasana.

Pranayama and Meditation This could be a short, guided practice or simply a few moments of silence for breath awareness and reflection.

3. Observe your students and identify which poses are causing them to struggle during the warm-up. Use these observations to adjust your class accordingly.

TIPS

» Be okay with everyone doing something slightly different, and support students in making wise choices for their bodies on that day.

» Offer personal time to help students one-on-one. Choose a pose to work on, set a timer, and walk around offering assistance.

CREATIVE SEQUENCING AND CUSTOMIZABLE VINYASA

Whether you're a yoga teacher looking for fresh ways to sequence your class or a home practitioner who wants to try something new, here are some of our favorite sequencing methods that go beyond the basic class blueprints.

THE ADD-ON METHOD

This sequencing method is great for yoga teachers who like to create fun, creative flows but don't want to overwhelm their students.

HOW IT WORKS: After your opening/warm-up, you practice a short sequence on one side, then the other. Then you repeat the sequence but add on a pose or two. Repeat the process until your sequence is complete, then flow through the whole thing once or twice before winding down with your cooldown and savasana.

BENEFITS: Because you move through many of the poses several times, this type of sequencing helps to build a sense of mastery. The familiarity of the repeated poses also makes it a good way to introduce a new pose or transition, and to offer options and variations without throwing too much information at students at once.

TYPES OF CLASSES IT WORKS BEST FOR: Vinyasa flow.

TIP Start small and avoid adding too much at once (just a pose or two each round is plenty). If you're a teacher, let your students know that they're going to have more than one opportunity to move through the sequence and that you'll add on a little each time. This removes the pressure that some students might feel to "get it right" from the get-go or to try the hardest/most "advanced" option every single time.

Here's a sample sequence:

Opening

» Take several mindful breaths in child's pose or crocodile pose.

Warm-up

» Downward-facing dog, moving around however you like.

» Walk forward to standing forward bend.

» Rise up and take one to two rounds of your favorite sun salute or other warm-up of choice.

Flow (Round 1)

» Chair pose

» Standing forward fold

» Step or jump back to a downward dog with your knees bent

» Lift your right leg up and step forward into a lunge on the right

» Step your left foot forward to meet your right and rise up into chair pose

» Switch sides

Flow (Round 2)

» Chair pose

» Standing forward fold

» Bent-knee downward dog

» Lift right leg up and step forward to lunge on the right

» Rise up into high lunge

» Warrior III

» Step left foot to meet right to return to chair pose

» Switch sides

Flow (Rounds 3 and 4)

» Chair pose

» Standing forward fold

» Bent-knee downward dog

» Lift right leg up and step forward to lunge on the right

» Rise up into a high lunge

» Warrior III

» Step back to lunge

» Open up into warrior II on the right

» Lower hands to the floor for low lunge on the right

» Step left foot forward to meet right, rise up to chair pose

» Switch sides

Cooldown

» From your final chair pose, lower down to seated

» Cow face pose on both sides

» Bound angle pose

» Savasana

THE HOLD-THEN-FLOW METHOD

As with the add-on method, this form of sequencing employs repetition in order to cultivate a sense of success.

HOW IT WORKS: After your opening and warm-up, do your sequence on both sides, spending some time in each pose (three to five breaths is a good starting place). Then, move through the same sequence again, this time "one-breath-per-movement style." Repeat a couple of times. Depending on your class length, you might go right into your cooldown after, or try the hold-then-flow method with another sequence.

BENEFITS: Often in vinyasa classes, we breeze right through poses. With the hold-then-flow method, you do (eventually) get to flow rapidly, but you also have the opportunity to spend a little more time with each pose. And here too, having the opportunity to repeat poses can take away the pressure to "get it right" the first time.

TYPES OF CLASSES IT WORKS BEST FOR: Vinyasa flow

TIP You can combine the hold-then-flow method with the add-on method: Teach the first part of your sequence, holding poses for three to five breaths each time. On your second round, move through the poses you already did one-breath-per-movement style, but hold the new poses you add on for three to five breaths. Continue like that until your sequence is complete, then flow through the whole thing, one breath per movement!

THE LET-THE-FATES-DECIDE METHOD

This sequencing method adds in the element of surprise, and is a great way to (literally) shake things up in a slower-paced class—in particular, one where you might be holding poses for a set period of time, or working on "skills and drills."

HOW IT WORKS: Grab a few paper lunch sacks or gift bags and label them with the specific pose or movement categories you want to offer in your class—for example, standing poses, balance poses, and core work. Write several different options on note cards that you place in the appropriate bags. After your warm-up, shake up your bags and let the fates decide what happens next! Pull an option from each bag, then repeat. The number of times you cycle through the bags will depend on your allotted class time, but be sure to include enough time at the end for a short cooldown and savasana.

You could even create a separate bag with cooldown options, such as bridge pose, pigeon, and supine twists!

BENEFITS: This type of sequencing can be fun for students and foster a sense of community—nothing brings folks together like a collective groan when the teacher pulls a one-minute plank hold out of the bag! It also takes the pressure off of teachers or home practitioners to always come up with something new. You can use the same bags several classes in a row and wind up with different sequences each time. You can also switch out some of the options every class to really keep things interesting!

TYPES OF CLASSES IT WORKS BEST FOR: Classes where you hold poses for some time such as hatha yoga classes focused on building stamina, Yin classes, and restorative classes. This method also works great for fusion and cross-training classes such as HIIT yoga classes.

TIP Make sure the poses and practices you include in your bags don't require a lot of specialized preparation. It's also a good idea to have a few bags you divide into categories (instead of just one bag). This way you won't accidentally end up with a class that's all warrior poses or all core work. And be specific! Write down hold times, breath cycles, or number of reps for each option, and keep the amount of time each option takes relatively consistent. If you're holding poses for time, it can be helpful to have a small timer on hand to keep track.

Here are some suggestions for poses you might include in a feel-good, stretch-focused class:

Bag 1: Lower-Body Stretches

» Pigeon pose (2 minutes on each side)

» Kneeling toe stretch (1 minute)

» Cow face pose (just the leg position, 2 minutes on each side)

» Head-to-knee pose (janu sirsasana) (2 minutes on each side)

» Fire log pose (2 minutes on each side)

Bag 2: Upper-Body Stretches and Backbends

» Cow face pose (just the arm position, sitting cross-legged or kneeling, 2 minutes on each side)

» Reclined hero (2 minutes)

» Supported bridge pose (2 minutes)

» Supine twist (2 minutes on each side)

Bag 3: Super-Relaxing Supine Poses

- » Legs-up-the-wall pose (2 minutes)
- » Reclined hand-to-big-toe pose wrapped in a strap (2 minutes on each side)
- » Simple reclined baby cradle variation (2 minutes on each side)
- » Revolved hand-to-big-toe pose

Here are some examples of poses and practices you might include in a strength- and stamina-focused class:

Bag 1: Standing Poses

- » Warrior II (1 minute on each side)
- » Chair pose at the wall (1 minute)
- » Half side-angle pose (30 seconds) into unsupported side-angle pose (30 seconds) (**Note:** you can also offer the option to hold half side-angle pose for the full 60 seconds)
- » Warrior III (1 minute on each side)
- » Goddess pose (1-minute hold with option to lift and lower one heel at a time)

Bag 2: Upper-Body Strength and Stamina Drills

- » Plank walks (lowering down to forearm plank then back up to plank, 30 seconds)
- » "Yoga push-ups" (elbows pointing back as in chaturanga, knees up or down, 30 seconds)
- » Classic push-ups (elbows wide, 30 seconds)
- » Triceps presses in reverse tabletop (Sit on the floor, knees bent, and place your hands behind you. Lift your hips to press up into a reverse tabletop position. Bend your elbows straight back, allowing your hips to lower a little, and then straighten your arms; 30 seconds)
- » Triceps presses from forearms and knees (come to forearms and knees, elbows stacked under shoulders, and lift your elbows away from the floor a little bit, pulsing them up and down without letting them touch the ground, 30 seconds)

Bag 3: Lower-Body Strength and Stamina Drills

- » Chair pose squats (coming in and out of chair pose) or jump squats (30 seconds)

- » Alternating lunges or "jump switch" lunges (30 seconds)

- » In the hands-and-knees position, hover knees away from the floor *just an inch* (30 seconds)

- » Goddess pose squats *or* jump back and forth from chair pose to goddess pose, like a "yoga jumping jack"

- » Bend and straighten both legs in a supported warrior III with hands on blocks and spine long (30 seconds on each side)

Bag 4: Core Work

- » Plank or forearm plank hold (1 minute)

- » Boat pose (1 minute)

- » Crunches with legs in baddha konasana, or bound angle, position

- » Oblique/bicycle crunches

- » "Superman" pose (prone, with legs, arms, and head lifted away from the floor, 1 minute)

17

Sample Sequences

Whether you have a few minutes or an hour, here are some of our favorite sequences. Try them, adapt them, share them. We hope they might inspire you to try something new—perhaps a transition, a variation with a prop, or a whole practice at the wall. The pose chapters share detailcd posc instructions you can refer back to if needed. You can try variations of any of these poses in any place! We haven't listed pranayama or meditation in these sequences, but we encourage you to try to incorporate these in your practice as well, to experience yoga more fully.

How long you hold the poses is up to you. Though we offer some suggestions, if you need more time in a pose, feel free to stay and explore the sensation, or stay for less time if that serves you best.

THE BASICS

This sequence keeps asana simple and accessible no matter where you are or how much time you have. It opens with a longer mountain pose to connect with your breath, the earth, and your power. Hold each pose for five to ten full breaths.

1. Mountain pose
2. Standing forward fold
3. Downward-facing dog
4. Plank
5. Downward-facing dog
6. Standing forward fold
7. High lunge (right)
8. Warrior II (right)
9. Extended side angle (right)
10. Downward-facing dog

    Repeat high lunge, warrior II, and extended side angle on the left
11. Downward-facing dog

    Rest in a child's pose, then lie on your back
12. Reclined twist
13. Reclined baby cradle variation
14. Legs-up-the-wall (5 minutes)

SUN SALUTATION WITH BLOCKS

We love teaching sun salutations with blocks to all levels of students—blocks can create a whole new experience of a familiar sequence! They can also add more space for transitions. Try the blocks at whatever height is comfortable. Work with your own pacing here. Try exploring one full breath with each movement, or hold each pose for a few breaths if you prefer.

1. Mountain pose
2. Forward fold or half forward fold with hands on blocks
3. Downward-facing dog with hands on blocks
4. Plank with hands on blocks
5. Chaturanga with hands on blocks
6. Upward-facing dog with hands on blocks
7. Downward-facing dog with hands on blocks
8. Forward fold with hands on blocks
9. Mountain pose

SUN SALUTATION WITH A CHAIR

You can use a chair to bring more stability into your sun salutations and to provide resistance as well. There are many ways to incorporate a chair in sun salutes; this variation is just one suggestion. Find a breath rhythm that works for you, either one breath per movement or holding each pose for a few breaths.

1. Mountain pose seated in chair
2. Forward fold seated in chair
3. Chair pose in or hovering above chair

   Stand up and turn the chair so the seat is facing you
4. Plank on chair
5. Chaturanga on chair
6. Upward-facing dog on chair
7. Downward-facing dog on chair

   Walk toward the chair to return to standing and then sit on the chair
8. Forward fold seated in chair
9. Chair pose in or hovering above chair
10. Mountain pose seated in chair

SUN SALUTATION AT THE WALL

Practicing sun salutations at the wall can offer practitioners of all levels a different experience of support. Here, too, you can go at a one-breath-per-movement pace or hold the poses longer.

1. Mountain pose facing the wall
2. Downward-facing dog at the wall
3. Crescent lunge at the wall (right)
4. Downward-facing dog at the wall
5. Crescent lunge at the wall (left)
6. Downward-facing dog at the wall
7. Plank to chaturanga at the wall
8. Upward-facing dog at the wall
9. Downward-facing dog at the wall
10. Mountain pose facing the wall

COMPLETE PRACTICE AT THE WALL

The wall is great for grounding poses and to help create balance in the postures. You can also use the wall for resistance in addition to support. Try holding each pose for five to ten breaths. It is okay to hold some poses longer than others.

1. Sun salutation at the wall
2. Chair pose at the wall
3. Warrior II at the wall with a block (both sides)
4. Triangle pose at the wall (both sides)
5. Warrior III at the wall (both sides)
6. Half moon pose at the wall (both sides)
7. Dolphin at the wall
8. Camel at the wall
9. Staff pose at the wall
10. A favorite twist, such as a supine spinal twist to wind down
11. Savasana or legs-up-the-wall (hold for as long as you like)

COMPLETE CHAIR PRACTICE

The use of the chair is great if you have limited mobility or are coming back from a long absence on the mat. The chair provides stability, comfort, and balance. The chair can also be challenging if you've never tried it. We encourage you to experiment with it! Try holding each pose five to ten breaths.

1. Sun salutation in a chair
2. Crescent lunge with a chair (both sides)
3. Goddess in, or hovering above, a chair
4. Warrior II in a chair (both sides)
5. Dolphin on a chair
6. Sugarcane bow on a chair (both sides)
7. Pigeon on a chair (both sides)
8. Downward-facing dog on a chair
9. Savasana, or legs-up-the-wall or on the seat of a chair (hold for as long as you like)

ARM-BALANCING WALL PRACTICE

The wall is a great prop for building confidence with arm balances. This sequence is challenging and tests your courage. Here we suggest beginning with your favorite sun salute variation or other warm-up. Planks and chaturangas can be particularly useful for preparing for arm balances, but don't do so many that your wrists are too tired for arm balances! Hold each pose for five to ten breaths.

Begin with a few rounds of your favorite sun-salute variation or other warm-up

1. Warrior II at the wall with a block
2. Half moon pose at the wall
3. L handstand at the wall
4. King Arthur pose (both sides; to open your hips, stretch your quads, and give your arms a reprieve)
5. Crow at the wall (you can also add side crow here)
6. Flying pigeon at the wall
7. Flying splits at the wall
8. Downward-facing dog at the wall
9. Bridge pose or other simple backbend of choice
10. Reclined twist
11. Legs-up-the-wall (hold for as long as you like)

CORE STRENGTH PRACTICE

Start by standing tall at the top of your mat, taking three to five breaths to begin. Feel your lower belly engage with every exhale, as though you were cinching a drawstring between your two frontal hip points. See if you can keep some of that engagement as you inhale, allowing the back and sides of your ribcage to expand. See if you can keep some of that expansion on your next exhale, reestablishing the engagement in your lower belly. Keep this focused breath with you as you move through the sequence.

1. Chair pose (hold five breaths or 30 seconds)
2. Standing forward bend
3. Plank or lower—one forearm at a time—to forearm plank (hold five breaths or 30 seconds)
4. Downward-facing dog
5. Crescent lunge
6. Warrior II
7. Half side-angle pose or extend your bottom foot for unsupported side-angle pose (hold for five breaths or 30 seconds)
8. Warrior II
9. Plank, or lower—one forearm at a time (leading with opposite forearm)—to forearm plank (hold for five breaths or 30 seconds)
10. Downward-facing dog

Repeat the standing-pose sequence on the left side

11. Plank (lower down onto your belly from here)
12. Cobra (inhale and rise to cobra three times, holding the last one for three to five breaths)
13. Downward-facing dog
14. Chair pose (lower down through your squat, or just sit down however you like to come into boat)
15. Boat pose or your favorite variation (hold for five breaths or 30 seconds)
16. Bridge pose (hold for five breaths or 30 seconds)
17. Savasana (3 minutes, or as long as you like)

HAPPY HIPS AND LEGS PRACTICE

This sequence is a great go-to after a run, walk, bike ride, or leg workout, or anytime you want to give your lower body some love. If you're craving some movement and/or standing poses before the static (held) stretches, after the kneeling toe stretch, do a few of your favorite warm-ups and/or sun salutations, and try a side angle pose (see page 82) for a few breaths on each side. Hold each pose five to ten breaths and hold savasana for as long as you like.

1. Kneeling toe stretch
2. Cow face pose
3. Fire log pose
4. Reclined hand-to-big-toe pose
5. Reclined baby cradle variation
6. Savasana

Recommended Resources

There are many wonderful classes and books available to help support your practice. Here are a few of our favorites.

ONLINE YOGA CLASSES

YOGA INTERNATIONAL (www.yogainternational.com)—we both have online classes in a variety of styles and focuses, and there are lots of other wonderful teachers you can practice with as well.

OMSTARS (www.omstars.com)—Dianne and other teachers share great classes here.

YOGA GIRL OFFICIAL (www.yogagirl.com)—Dianne and other teachers share a variety great classes here as well.

DIANNE BONDY YOGA ONLINE (yogaforeveryone.tv and YouTube, search Dianne Bondy)— short sequences and reflections every Friday, all free, many focused on accessibility!

BOOKS

Bacon, Linda. *Health at Every Size: The Surprising Truth about Your Weight*. Dallas: BenBella, 2010.

Baker, Jes. *Landwhale: On Turning Insults into Nicknames, Why Body Image Is Hard, and How Diets Can Kiss My Ass*. New York: Seal, 2018.

———. *Things No One Will Tell Fat Girls: A Handbook for Unapologetic Living*. New York: Seal, 2015.

Bondy, Dianne. *Yoga for Everyone: 50 Poses for Every Type of Body*. New York: Alpha, 2019.

Clark, Bernie. *Your Body, Your Yoga: Learn Alignment Cues That Are Skillful, Safe, and Best Suited to You*. Wild Strawberry, 2016.

———. *Your Spine, Your Yoga: Developing Stability and Mobility for Your Spine*. Wild Strawberry, 2018.

Guest-Jelley, Anna. *Curvy Yoga: Love Yourself & Your Body a Little More Each Day*. New York: Sterling, 2017.

Guest-Jelley, Anna, and Melanie C. Klein. *Yoga and Body Image: 25 Personal Stories about Beauty, Bravery & Loving Your Body*. Woodbury, MN: Llewellyn, 2014.

Heagberg, Kat, Kathryn Ashworth, Melanie C. Klein, and Toni Willis. *Embodied Resilience through Yoga: 30 Mindful Essays about Finding Empowerment after Addiction, Trauma, Grief, and Loss*. Woodbury, MN: Llewellyn, 2020.

Heyman, Jivana. *Accessible Yoga: Poses and Practices for Every Body*. Boulder: Shambhala, 2019.

Johnson, Michelle C. *Skill in Action: Radicalizing Your Yoga Practice to Create a Just World*. Radical Transformation Media, 2017.

Klein, Melanie C. *Yoga Rising: 30 Empowering Stories from Yoga Renegades for Every Body*. Woodbury, MN: Llewellyn, 2018.

Mitchell, Jules. *Yoga Biomechanics: Stretching Redefined*. Scotland, UK: Handspring, 2019.

Sanford, Matthew. *Waking: A Memoir of Trauma and Transcendence*. Emmaus, PA: Rodale, 2008.

Sell, Christina. *Yoga from the Inside Out: Making Peace with Your Body through Yoga*. Chino Valley, AZ: Hohm, 2003.

Spindler, Beth. *Yoga Therapy for Fear: Treating Anxiety, Depression and Rage with the Vagus Nerve and Other Techniques*. Philadelphia: Singing Dragon, 2018.

Stanley, Jessamyn. *Every Body Yoga: Let Go of Fear, Get On the Mat, Love Your Body*. New York: Workman, 2017.

Meet the Models

Yoga is for everyone, and the models demonstrating the poses in this book range from beginner to experienced yoga practitioners.

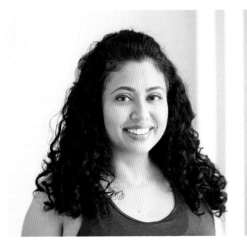

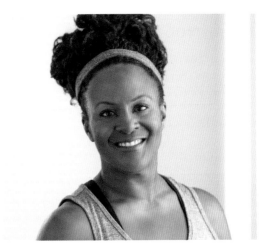

DEEPALI

How long have you been practicing yoga?
I have been practicing for seven years.

What does yoga mean to you?
To me, yoga means self-healing, self-help, expansion, elevation . . . a toolkit to navigate this journey called life.

Favorite pose?
I can only pick one?! My go-to is cat/cow and all its variations.

Least favorite pose?
Frog.

What inspires you to practice?
The mind-body-spirit connection that I feel when I practice yoga is what inspires me to do it daily.

How do you make your practice your own?
I make my practice my own by honoring myself and where I'm at that day or that moment. I focus on how it feels inside, rather than how it looks on the outside.

DIANNE

How long have you been practicing yoga?
A long, long time! On and off for most of my life.

What does yoga mean to you?
Yoga to me means self-preservation, action, and self-reflection. Yoga is the ability to be skillful at life and take action for change.

Favorite pose?
Triangle.

Least favorite pose?
Flying splits.

What inspires you to practice?
I love how powerful it makes me feel, how it clears my mind, relieves my anxiety, and how it inspires me to appreciate my body.

How do you make your practice your own?
I have a dedicated space in my home. I remind myself every day that I am worth taking time for. I have the privilege to exist in this body and I do all I can to honor it

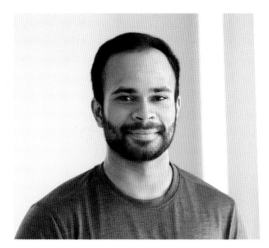

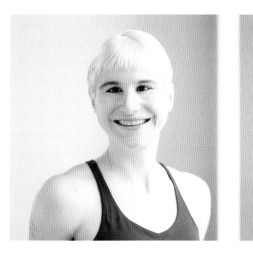

JAI

How long have you been practicing yoga?
I have been practicing at the beginner level for about a year—since I started working as a videographer and video editor for Yoga International.

What does yoga mean to you?
To me, yoga is a way to decompress both mentally and physically.

Favorite pose?
Child's pose or savasana.

Least favorite pose?
Pigeon pose.

What inspires you to practice?
I'm inspired by seeing how much other people enjoy practicing and being part of the yoga community.

How do you make your practice your own?
I make my practice my own by knowing my limits and practicing poses I enjoy while not forcing myself into poses that aren't accessible to me.

KAT

How long have you been practicing yoga?
I took my first yoga class on my first day of college when I was seventeen years old (which, at the time I'm writing this, was almost fifteen years ago). I started teaching when I was nineteen and have been at it ever since!

What does yoga mean to you?
For me, yoga is a way to be with myself, even when being with myself is challenging. It's something in my day that's always there, always consistent, no matter where I am in the world, even if it's just for ten minutes. It's a practice that can grow as I grow. And it's also a lot of fun!

Favorite pose?
Handstand!

Least favorite pose?
Wheel pose.

What inspires you to practice?
Remembering how good I'll feel after inspires me to practice. I've never once regretted rolling out my yoga mat.

CONTINUED ▶

How do you make your practice your own?
I make my practice my own by adapting poses to fit my needs and goals, by exploring new pose variations, and also by incorporating different forms of movement into my practice. Before I was a yoga practitioner I was a dancer, and I taught Pilates and group fitness for a while too, so I enjoy bringing movement from other modalities onto my mat from time to time.

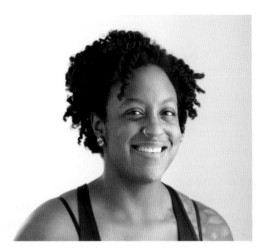

KIANA

How long have you been practicing yoga?
I was originally introduced to yoga classes when I was fourteen, but my practice became really consistent around the time I started my 200-hour teacher training in Texas. I finished training in May 2017.

What does yoga mean to you?
I see yoga as a lifelong practice of self-study and self-love that has no expectations to be met and no room for self-condemnation. Yoga means personal time with yourself, giving yourself space to breathe, to move because it feels good.

Favorite pose?
Dolphin pose and forearm balance. They remind me of my inner strength, and there are so many fun variations!

Least favorite pose?
I could probably do without pigeon. It gets the right muscles and I appreciate the stretch after work, but only for about five seconds (if I can even last that long).

What inspires you to practice?
Practicing consistently means I can be the best version of myself: the version who lives to support those around me and to support nature, which provides everything we need. If I practice regularly, I create an extra capacity to study and share therapeutic yoga techniques. It also reminds me to spend time in nature daily and to take extra steps to reduce my carbon footprint.

How do you make your practice your own?
Creating a lifestyle out of yoga has worked best for me—from doing asanas at work to applying Ayurvedic tips for meals and wellness. Taking the practice off of the mat, by improving how I interact with others and transforming deep-seated habits and thought patterns is where the real work is for me.

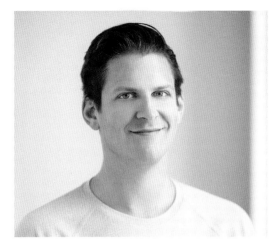

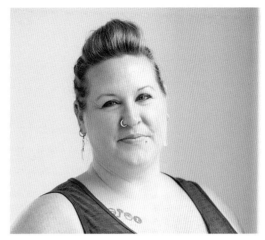

KYLE

How long have you been practicing yoga?
I've been practicing yoga for about seven years.

What does yoga mean to you?
It's complicated . . .

Favorite pose?
Shoulderstand!

Least favorite pose?
Anything that requires bearing weight through my hands and wrists.

What inspires you to practice?
I will almost always show up for a yoga class in an unconventional space with live music!

How do you make your practice your own?
I will sometimes incorporate vinyasa flows into weird performance art pieces. Otherwise, I use mountains of blocks!

PAGE

How long have you been practicing yoga?
I've done yoga sporadically for the past ten years or so, but my practice has become much more consistent this past year.

What does yoga mean to you?
Yoga means a place to let go of all the distractions and connect my mind, body, and spirit.

Favorite pose?
Warrior II.

Least favorite pose?
Frog.

What inspires you to practice?
The continued strength, alignment, and guidance that yoga brings me.

How do you make your practice your own?
Every time I come to the mat I take a moment to align my body and mind and to set my intention for that specific practice.

Notes

1. "History of Kemetic Yoga," www.kemeticyoga.com/history-of-kemetic-yoga.

2. "About Yirser Ra Hotep," www.kemeticyoga.com/what-is-kemetic-yoga /about-yirser-ra-hotep.

3. "About Yirser Ra Hotep."

4. David Gordon White, "Yoga, Brief History of an Idea," in *Yoga in Practice*, ed. David Gordon White (Princeton University Press, 2012), http://assets.press .princeton.edu/chapters/i9565.pdf.

5. White, "Yoga, Brief History of an Idea."

6. Amy Roeder, "America Is Failing Its Black Mothers," *Harvard Public Health Magazine*, Winter 2019, www.hsph.harvard.edu/magazine/magazine_article /america-is-failing-its-black-mothers.

7. John LaRosa, "Top 9 Things to Know about the Weight Loss Industry," *Market Research* (blog), March 6, 2019, www.blog.marketresearch.com/u.s.-weight-loss -industry-grows-to-72-billion.

8. Deborah A. Christel, "Average American Women's Clothing Size: Comparing National Health and Nutritional Examination Surveys (1988–2010) to ASTM International Misses & Women's Plus Size Clothing," *International Journal of Fashion Design, Technology and Education* 10, no. 2 (2017): 129–36.

9. Charles Manning and Tara Rice, "What If Runway Models Were the Size of an Average American Woman?" *Cosmopolitan*, February 18, 2015, www.cosmopolitan .com/style-beauty/fashion/a36687/runway-models-average-size-american-woman/.

10. Judith Rodin, Lisa Silberstein, and Ruth Striegel Weissman, "Women and Weight: A Normative Discontent," *Nebraska Symposium on Motivation* 32 (February 1984): 267–307.

11. Mario Palmer, "5 Facts about Body Image," *Amplify* via DoSomething.org, February 24, 2014, www.dosomething.org/us/facts/11-facts-about-body-image.

12. "Survey Finds That Women Are More Likely to Consider Plastic Surgery Than They Were Ten Years Ago," The American Society for Aesthetic Plastic Surgery, 2014, www.dosomething.org/us/facts/11-facts-about-body-image.

13. Palmer, "5 Facts about Body Image."

14. *Anjaneyasana* is named for the mythical monkey god Hanuman, who also goes by the name Anjaneya, which means "son of Anjana" (Anjana being his mother).

Index

About the Authors

DIANNE BONDY is a celebrated yoga teacher, social justice activist, and leading voice of the Yoga for All movement. Her inclusive view of yoga asana and philosophy inspires and empowers thousands of followers around the world—regardless of their shape, size, ethnicity, or level of ability. Dianne contributes to Yoga International, Yoga Girl, Do You Yoga, and Omstars, and is the author of the book *Yoga for Everyone: 50 Poses for Every Type of Body*. She has been featured in publications such as the *Guardian*, *Huffington Post*, *Cosmopolitan*, and *People*.

KAT HEAGBERG is editor-in-chief of Yoga International and has been teaching yoga regularly since 2005. Her Yoga International video classes and workshops are consistently among the top viewed each month. She's also a host of the *Yoga Talk* podcast and co-editor of the book *Embodied Resilience through Yoga*.